OXFORD MEDICAL PUBLICATIONS

Oxford Handbook of
Reproductive Medicine and Family Planning

Published and forthcoming Oxford Handbooks

Oxford Handbook of Clinical Medicine 7/e (also available for PDAs)
Oxford Handbook of Clinical Specialties 7/e
Oxford Handbook of Acute Medicine 2/e
Oxford Handbook of Anaesthesia 2/e
Oxford Handbook of Applied Dental Sciences
Oxford Handbook of Cardiology
Oxford Handbook of Clinical Dentistry 4/e
Oxford Handbook of Clinical and Laboratory Investigation 2/e
Oxford Handbook of Clinical Diagnosis
Oxford Handbook of Clinical Haematology 2/e
Oxford Handbook of Clinical Immunology and Allergy 2/e
Oxford Handbook of Clinical Pharmacy
Oxford Handbook of Clinical Surgery 3/e
Oxford Handbook of Critical Care 2/e
Oxford Handbook of Dental Patient Care 2/e
Oxford Handbook of Dialysis 2/e
Oxford Handbook of Emergency Medicine 3/e
Oxford Handbook of Endocrinology and Diabetes
Oxford Handbook of ENT and Head and Neck Surgery
Oxford Handbook for the Foundation Programme
Oxford Handbook of Gastroenterology and Hepatology
Oxford Handbook of General Practice 2/e
Oxford Handbook of Genitourinary Medicine, HIV and AIDS
Oxford Handbook of Geriatric Medicine
Oxford Handbook of Medical Sciences
Oxford Handbook of Nephrology and Hypertension
Oxford Handbook of Nutrition and Dietetics
Oxford Handbook of Neurology
Oxford Handbook of Occupational Health
Oxford Handbook of Obstetrics and Gynaecology
Oxford Handbook of Oncology 2/e
Oxford Handbook of Ophthalmology
Oxford Handbook of Palliative Care
Oxford Handbook of Practical Drug Therapy
Oxford Handbook of Pre-Hospital Care
Oxford Handbook of Psychiatry
Oxford Handbook of Public Health Practice 2/e
Oxford Handbook of Rehabilitation Medicine
Oxford Handbook of Respiratory Medicine
Oxford Handbook of Rheumatology 2/e
Oxford Handbook of Sport and Exercise Medicine
Oxford Handbook of Tropical Medicine 2/e
Oxford Handbook of Urology

Oxford Handbook of
Reproductive Medicine and Family Planning

Enda McVeigh
Senior Fellow in Reproductive Medicine
University of Oxford, UK

Professor Roy Homburg
Head of Division of Reproductive Medicine
Department of Obstetrics and Gynaecology
VU Medical Centre
Amsterdam
The Netherlands

Professor John Guillebaud
Emeritus Professor of Family Planning and
Reproductive Health
University College London, UK

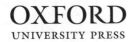

OXFORD
UNIVERSITY PRESS

OXFORD
UNIVERSITY PRESS

Great Clarendon Street, Oxford OX2 6DP

Oxford University Press is a department of the University of Oxford.
It furthers the University's objective of excellence in research, scholarship,
and education by publishing worldwide in

Oxford New York

Auckland Cape Town Dar es Salaam Hong Kong Karachi
Kuala Lumpur Madrid Melbourne Mexico City Nairobi
New Delhi Shanghai Taipei Toronto

With offices in

Argentina Austria Brazil Chile Czech Republic France Greece
Guatemala Hungary Italy Japan Poland Portugal Singapore
South Korea Switzerland Thailand Turkey Ukraine Vietnam

Oxford is a registered trade mark of Oxford University Press
in the UK and in certain other countries

Published in the United States
by Oxford University Press Inc., New York

© Oxford University Press, 2008

The moral rights of the authors have been asserted
Database right Oxford University Press (maker)

First published 2008

British Library Cataloguing in Publication Data
Data available

Library of Congress Cataloging in Publication Data
Data available

Typeset by Newgen Imaging Systems (P) Ltd., Chennai, India
Printed in Italy
on acid-free paper by
Lego Print S.p.A

ISBN 978-0-19-920380-2 (flexicover: alk.paper)

10 9 8 7 6 5 4 3 2 1

Foreword

Reproductive Medicine in the twenty-first century is an exciting and fast evolving field which sits as one of the subspecialties of Obstetrics and Gynaecology, but which has evolved to have an important multi-professional dimension, which includes embryology and andrology, nursing, endocrinology, social science, and basic reproductive sciences, as well as practical ethics and law.

Thirty years ago, when I entered the field, the topics covered here might all have been represented in a textbook, but the subject would have been labelled as Gynaecological Endocrinology, or just Gynaecology. What has changed is the explosion in understanding and in the treatment possibilities for which the development of assisted reproductive technologies and endoscopic surgery have been transformational. The explosion has not been restricted to the clinical field. The unprecedented access to the ovary and to early human development has made possible a rapid expansion of our biological understanding, and when this is combined with the expanded horizons provided by reproductive and stem cell technologies developed in animal species, the scientific perspective has matured rapidly. The scale and diversity of reproductive medicine is now such that most practitioners would not expect to encompass all of the topic areas in their routine practice, but it is important that the coherence of Reproductive Medicine is presented in textbook form for the benefit of trainees and others, from whatever background, who need to understand the scope and diversity of the field.

The title of this handbook separates out Family Planning for mention as a separate topic, but in many ways it is an integral component of Reproductive Medicine. In practical terms the separate labelling is justified on the basis that there is a significant community who practice within Family Planning and Reproductive Healthcare, who do not generally practice more widely in Reproductive Medicine, just as many in Reproductive Medicine do not practice widely in Family Planning. Both groups can benefit from a good overview of the whole of the field and the title sends that signal to both groups.

In this handbook readers will find coverage of the whole spectrum. It is logical that the developmental genetic factors and the structural development of the reproductive tract and its abnormalities is the starting point for this text, leading into an overview of the basics of the biochemistry relevant to reproduction. With this scene set the authors have surveyed the topic areas in a sequential fashion, following the female life cycle from menarche and disorders of adolescence, through chapters covering the ovarian cycle and menstruation. This latter subject is followed by the associated functional abnormalities, both of menstrual pattern and intensity, as well as associated problems linked to androgens. Finally, in the coverage of the female life cycle, there is the menopause and its management. The substantial subsequent coverage is in two important topic areas, infertility and family planning, each of which is covered under a range of appropriate chapters.

In my years as Editor-in-Chief of the journal *Human Reproduction* I sought to ensure that we encompassed all aspects of the field, and I am pleased to see that the authors here have taken the same approach. With increasing specialization and fragmentation of the field, there will be many who see their horizon as infertility and assisted reproduction, whereas others might practice mainly in endometriosis and pain, or in the post-reproductive area on the menopause and HRT. It is important that all have a broad knowledge of the whole field, since the implications of our findings and interventions may well be wider than our sub-subspecialty area. This Oxford Handbook well serves the purpose of providing a good overview of its subject for student and specialist alike, presented by authors of international reputation.

Professor David H Barlow
Executive Dean of Medicine and Professor of Reproductive Medicine
The University of Glasgow

Authors' disclaimer and statement of competing interests

This book represents the personal opinions of the authors, based wherever possible on published and sometimes unpublished evidence. When (as is not infrequent) no epidemiological or other direct evidence is available, clinical advice herein is always as practical and realistic as possible and based, pending more data, on the authors' judgement of other sources. These may include the opinions of Expert Committees and any existing Guidelines. In some instances the advice appearing in this book may even so differ appreciably from the latter, for reasons usually given in the text and (since medical knowledge and practice are continually evolving) relates to the date of publication. Healthcare professionals must understand that they take ultimate responsibility for their patient and ensure that any clinical advice they use from this book is applicable to the specific circumstances that they encounter.

Statement of competing interests

The authors have received payments for research projects, lectures, *ad hoc* consultancy work and related expenses from the manufacturers of pharmaceutical products.

EM
RH
JG

Contents

Part 2: Contraception and Family Planning

Detailed contents

Symbols and abbreviations

1°	secondary
2°	primary
±	plus or minus
☙	controversial topic
📖	page number in this volume
ABP	androgen-binding protein
ACTH	adrenocorticotrophic hormone
AFS	American Fertility Society
ALO	Actinomyces-like organisms
AMH	anti-Mullerian hormone
AMI	acute myocardial infarction
BBD	benign breast disease
BBT	basal body temperature
BMI	body mass index
BNF	British National Formulary
BP	blood pressure
BTB	breakthrough bleeding
CAH	congenital adrenal hyperplasia
CAIS	complete androgen insensitivity syndrome
CBG	corticosteroid-binding globulin
CC	clomifene citrate
CGHFBC	Collaborative Group on Hormonal Factors in Breast Cancer
CHD	coronary heart disease
CIN	cervical intraepithelial neoplasia
CNS	central nervous system
COC	combined oral contraception/ive
COEC	combined oral emergency contraceptive
CPA	cyproterone acetate
CRH	corticotrophin-releasing hormone
CSM	Committee on the Safety of Medicines (UK)
CT	computed tomography
CVS	cardiovascular system
DES	diethylstilboestrol
DFFP	Diploma of the Faculty of Family Planning and Reproductive Health Care
DHEAS	dehydroepiandrosterone sulfate
DHT	dihydrotestosterone

DM	diabetes mellitus
DMPA	depot medroxyprogesterone acetate
DNA	deoxyribonucleic acid
DoH	Department of Health (now termed DH)
DSG	desogestrel
DSP	drospirenone
EC	emergency contraception
EE	ethinylestradiol
EID	enzyme inducer drug
ET	embryo transfer
EVA	ethylene vinyl acetate
FFPRHC	Faculty of Family Planning and Reproductive Health
FAQ	frequently asked question
FERC	frozen embryo replacement cycle
FGD 2003	Faculty Guidance Document 2003
FPA	Family Planning Association
FSH	follicle-stimulating hormone
GBG	gonadal steroid-binding globulin
GIFT	gamete intrafallopian tube transfer
GnRH	gonadotrophin-releasing hormone
GSD	gestodene
GUM	Genitourinary Medicine
hCG	human chorionic gonadotrophin
HDL	high-density lipoprotein
HFEA	Human Fertilization and Embryology Authority
HIV	human immunodeficiency virus
hMG	human menopausal gonadotrophin
HMG	high mobility group
HPV	human papillomavirus
HRT	hormone replacement therapy
HS	haemorrhagic stroke
HSG	hysterosalpingography
5-HT	5-hydroxytryptamine
HUS	haemolytic uraemic syndrome
ICSI	intracytoplasmic sperm injection
i.m.	intramuscular
INR	international normalized ratio—blood test used to control warfarin anticoagulant level
IPPF	International Planned Parenthood Federation
IS	ischaemic stroke
IUD	intra-uterine device
IUI	intra-uterine insemination
IUS	intra-uterine system

i.v.	intravenous
IVF	in vitro fertilization
LAM	lactational amenorrhoea method
LARC	long-acting reversible contraceptive
LCR	ligase chain reaction—ultrasensitive and specific test (e.g. for Chlamydia)
LDL	low-density lipoprotein
LH	luteinizing hormone
LNG	levonorgestrel
LOCAH	late-onset congenital adrenal hyperplasia
LOD	laparoscopic ovarian drilling
MAR	mixed antibody reaction
MFFP	Membership of the Faculty of Family Planning and Reproductive Health Care
MHRA	Medicines and Healthcare Products Regulatory Agency
MIS	Mullerian-inhibiting substance
MPA	medroxyprogesterone acetate
MRI	magnetic resonance imaging
MRKH	Mayer–Rokitansky–Kuster–Hauser
NET	norethisterone (termed norethindrone in the USA)
NETA	norethisterone acetate
NFP	natural family planning
NGM	norgestimate
NICE	National Institute for Health and Clinical Excellence
OHSS	ovarian hyperstimulation syndrome
OR	odds ratio
PCOS	polycystic ovarian syndrome
PCR	polymerase chain reaction (like LCR, for ultrasensitive/specific tests)
PCT	postcoital test
PFI	pill-free interval
PID	pelvic inflammatory disease
PIL	Patient Information Leaflet
PKC	protein kinase C
PMS	premenstrual syndrome
POEC	progestogen-only emergency contraceptive
POP	progestogen-only pill
RCGP	Royal College of General Practitioners
RCN	Royal College of Nursing
RCOG	Royal College of Obstetricians and Gynaecologists
RCT	randomized controlled trial
s.c.	subcutaneous
SHGB	sex hormone-binding globulin

SLE	systemic lupus erythematosus
SPC	Summary of Product Characteristics (= Data Sheet)
SRE	sex and relationships education
STD	sexually transmitted disease
STI	sexually transmitted infection
TGF	transforming growth factor
TIA	transient ischaemic attack
TSH	thyroid-stimulating hormone
TTP	thrombotic thrombocytopenic purpura
TVS	transvaginal scanning
UKMEC	adaptation of WHO's Medical Eligibility Criteria for Faculty of FP – Contraceptive Use
UPSI	unprotected sexual intercourse
VTE	venous thromboembolism
VV	varicose veins
WHI	Women's Health Initiative
WHO	World Health Organization
WHOMEC	WHO Medical Eligibility Criteria for contraceptive use
WHOSPR	WHO's Selected Practice Recommendations for contraceptive use

Part I

Reproductive Medicine

Sexual differentiation

Key stages of fetal sex differentiation

Genetic sex is determined at the moment of conception by the presence or absence of the Y chromosome, and after week 6 of fetal life it will guide the subsequent development of the fetus down one of two standard pathways—male or female (see figure 1.1).

- Week 3: primordial germ cells present in the endoderm of the yolk sac.
- Week 5–6: germs cells migrate to the genital ridge (future gonad).
- Week 6: primitive sex cords form around the germ cells; two Mullerian (or paramesonephric) ducts lateral to the Wolffian (or mesonephric) ducts.
- Week 6: the cloacal membrane at the caudal end of the fetus separates into the anterior urogenital and posterior anal parts.
- Week 7: the urogenital section of the cloacal membrane, the genital tubercle, urogenital folds, and lateral and labioscrotal swelling will differentiate into the future external genitalia.

After gonadal differentiation has occurred, the presence or absence of gonadal hormone production and other fetal factors then guides the development of the Mullerian ducts, Wolffian ducts and external genitalia. The testes secrete androgens, leading to male external genital development and differentiation of the bilateral Wolffian ducts into the vas deferens, seminal vesicle and epididymis. The testes also secrete anti-Mullerian hormone (AMH—also know as Mullerian-inhibiting substance, MIS), leading to the regression of the Mullerian ducts. The fetal ovaries do not secrete androgens or AMH and therefore the female external genital development, growth of the Mullerian ducts and spontaneous regression of the Wolffian ducts occur.

- Gonads undifferentiated until 7–8 weeks of gestation.
- Associated with a dual ductal system.
- Mesonephric ducts form first.
- At 6 weeks, paramesonephric ducts form lateral to the mesonephric ducts.
- Mesonephric ducts degenerate.
- Mullerian ducts form.
  - Cranial ends become fallopian tubes.
  - Caudal ends fuse to form the uterus.
- By ~9 weeks a uterine cervix is visible.
- By 17 weeks myometrium is formed.

Week 6   Week 9

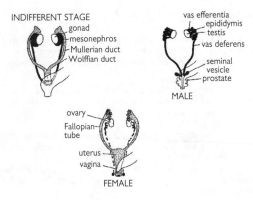

Fig.1.1 Key satges of fetal Sex differentiation.

The SRY gene

The presence or absence of the SRY gene (sex-determining region of the Y chromosome) at the end of week 6 of fetal development will guide the indifferent gonad to commence development into an ovary or testis.

Key facts about the SRY gene
- High mobility group (HMG) box family of DNA-binding proteins.
- Master control gene for testis determination.
- DNA/RNA-binding protein.
- Molecular targets unknown.
- Precipitates cascade of gene expression required for testis formation.
- Expression is transiently activated in a centre-to-pole wave along the anteroposterior (AP) axis of developing XY gonads.
- Shortly after the onset of *Sry* activation, *Sox9* (*Sry*-related HMG box-9) is also activated in a centre-to-pole pattern similar to the initial *Sry* expression profile.

Other genes involved in sex determination

There are two other genes, DMRT-1 and DAX-1, that are involved in sex determination in the developing fetus:

DMRT-1

- Chromosome 9 transcription factor.
- Critical in human sex determination—expressed in genital ridges and in Sertoli cells. Increases during testis development and decreases in ovary.
- Mutations in this region are associated with male to female sex reversal.
- DMT1-related sequences have also been found in the chick, alligator and mouse.
- DMRT genes are expressed only in the genital ridges of male embryos.

DAX-1

- Chromosome X p21.3–p21.2 nuclear receptor family.
- Expressed in both gonadal ridges then persists in the ovary and decreases in the testis according to switch on of *Sry*.
- Anti-testis gene by acting antagonistically to *Sry*?
- Responsible for **DSS syndrome** (dosage-sensitive sex reversal). Dosage-sensitive sex reversal is due to duplication of the gene in humans.

Abnormal embryological development—intersex conditions

Intersex is defined as a mix or blend of the physically defining features associated with the male or females, i.e. karyotype, gonadal structure, internal genitalia and external genitalia. Most intersex conditions occur due to a genetic or environmental disruption to the pathway of fetal sexual development. This disruption can be to gonadal differentiation or development, sex steroid production, sex steroid conversion or tissue utilization of sex steroid.

Incidence

The estimated incidence in the UK is 1 in 2000. Conditions with autosomal recessive inheritance are more common in populations where intermarriage is common.

Presentation and investigation

Each intersex condition has a spectrum of severity and therefore may present in a variety of ways:

> Ambiguous genitalia.
> Salt-losing crisis in neonatal life (congenital adrenal hyperplasia).
> Pelvic mass with gonadal tumour.
> Inguinal hernia with unexpected gonad.
> Ambiguity of the genitalia developing in childhood or puberty.
> Sibling history of intersex.
> Primary amenorrhoea or puberty delay.
> Infertility.
> Sexual dysfunction.

Initial investigation with depend on the presentation but should include:

Initial	Further investigations
Karyotype	Androstendione
Testosterone and oestradiol	Dihydrotestosterone (DHT)
Luteinizing hormone (LH) and follicle-stimulating hormone (FSH)	24h urine for steroid metabolites
17-Hydroxyprogesterone	Synacthen test
Pelvic imaging—ultrasound or MRI	Renal ultrasound

Management of intersex conditions

The management of these conditions will depend on acquiring an accurate diagnosis and then the referral on to an appropriate paediatric or adult multidisciplinary team (endocrinology, gynaecology, surgery and psychology). Areas that they will have to consider will include:

- Need for hormone replacement.
- Screening for associated medical conditions.
- Psychological treatment.
- Genetic counselling for other family members.
- Sex assignment for children.
- Gonadal malignancy risk.
- Fertility options.
- Genital surgery options for ambiguous genitalia.
- Vaginal enlargement options.
- Assess to peer support.

The disorders can be categorized into three main areas: gonadal dysgenesis (complete and partial), hermaphroditism (true/primary and pseudo/secondary) and dysgenesis of the uterus, vagina and external genitalia.

Complete (pure) gonadal dysgenesis. This is due to a 1° defect in gonadal formation. The karyotype may be a normal 46, XX or 46, XY. Little is known about the 46, XX condition apart from the fact that some have homozygous FSH receptor mutations, also seen in males when they have impaired spermatogenesis. In the 46, XY condition, 20% have lesions in the SRY gene while the remainder have the abnormalities in the X chromosome or autosomes. In these cases, gonadal development is arrested **before** MIS (AMH) and androgens are produced. This results in the formation of bilateral streak gonads associated with an immature female phenotype. There are no other associated somatic defects. The result clinically is a delayed puberty and amenorrhoea which is oestrogen responsive.

Complete gonadal dysgenesis. This condition is also the result of a 1° defect in gonadal formation, but in these cases there are bilateral streak gonads. Typically the karotype is 45, XO Turner's syndrome, and all have partial or complete loss of material from an X chromosome. It occurs in 1 in 2500 live births. Somatic defects are present in these cases and include: facial dystrophy, short stature and renal anomalies. There is again a delay in puberty which is oestrogen responsive. Fertility is rare but is reported more in cases of mosaicism.

Mixed gonadal dysgenesis. This occurs in mosaics: 46, XY or 45 XO; 46, XY. It results in unilateral testis and contralateral streak gonad. There is persistence of the Mullerian duct structures, the vagina and uterus, and most have a fallopian tube on the side of the streak. The external genitalia are ambiguous. In the case of XY, they are undervirilized.

Hermaphroditism

Hermaphroditism is defined as 'true' in cases where there is both an ovary and testis or an ovotestis, or pseudohermaphrodite (male) where there are two testes and pseudohermaphrodite (female) where there are two ovaries. The most common karyotype in true hermaphroditism is 46, XX. Ovarian and testicular tissues can be present, separately or as an ovotestis. The external genitalia tend to be masculinized.

Secondary or pseudohermaphrodites

(XY) Testicular feminization *or* **androgen insensitivity syndrome** (complete = testis + female soma. Population incidence 0.005%; partial = poorly developed male soma. Population incidence 0.01%). Defect in androgen receptor or androgen synthesis. They have MIS and so no Mullerian ducts or associated structures develop. In complete androgen insensitivity syndrome (CAIS), there can be completely normal external genitalia. Absent **or** rudimentary Wolffian duct derivatives. Absence or presence of epididymides and/or vas deferens. Inguinal **or** labial testes; short blind-ending vagina.

(XX) Congenital adrenohyperplasia or adrenogenital syndrome (ovary + variable somatic maleness: partial has population incidence of 1%, complete 0.01%). 21-Hydroxylase deficiency is the most common autosomal recessive genetic disorder. The most common cause of genital ambiguity of the newborn in the UK. The genitalia can range from clitoral enlargement to complete labioscrotal fusion and a penile urethra. The size and entry level of vagina into the urogenital sinus is abnormal. There are normal internal Mullerian duct derivatives. An increase in androgens can be seen as early as 7–8 weeks of fetal life, but there is no MIS.

(XY) 5-alpha-reductase deficiency: 46, XY with normal testes but lacking the enzyme in external genitalia and urogenital sinus, and unable to make DHT. Minimally virilized at birth then extreme virilization at puberty.

Mullerian anomalies

Abnormal development of the Mullerian ducts can lead to a wide range of conditions (see figure 1.3). Many are subtle variations of normal Mullerian anatomy and often remain asymptomatic or require no treatment. Others are transverse or longitudinal structures and may present in a variety of ways. An understanding of the timing and sequence of embryological development of the entire urogenital system helps in understanding the conditions (see figure 1.2).

- Vaginal development begins at 9 weeks.
- Uterovaginal plate forms between the caudal buds of the Mullerian ducts and dorsal wall of the urogenital sinus.
- Upper 1/3 of vagina develops from paramesonephric ducts.
- Remainder from urogenital sinus.

Mullerian anomalies—The American Fertility Society (AFS) classification

The classification most used to list Mullerian anomalies is that of the American Fertility Society. Congenital Mullerian abnormalities generally fall into one of three groups: a normally fused single Mullerian system with agenesis of one or more parts; a unicornuate system (unilateral hypoplasia or agenesis of one Mullerian dust); or lateral fusion failures (including didelphic and bicornuate anomalies). Complete agenesis is separated in Rokitansky syndrome (also called Mayer–Rokitansky–Kuster–Hauser (MRKH) syndrome).

- **Class I (hypoplasia/agenesis)**: uterine/cervical agenesis or hypoplasia. MRKH syndrome—combined agenesis of the uterus, cervix and upper portion of the vagina.
- **Class II (unicornuate uterus)**: a unicornuate uterus is the result of complete, or almost complete, arrest of development of one Mullerian duct. Incomplete in 90% of patients.
- **Class III (didelphic uterus)**: complete non-fusion of both Mullerian ducts. The individual horns are fully developed and almost normal in size. Two cervices.
- **Class IV (bicornuate uterus)**: partial non-fusion of the Mullerian ducts.
- **Class V (septate uterus)**: a septate uterus results from failure of resorption of the septum between the two uterine horns. The septum can be partial or complete.
- **Class VI (arcuate uterus)**: an arcuate uterus has a single uterine cavity with a convex or flat uterine fundus.
- **Class VII (diethylstilboestrol (DES)-related anomaly)**:
  - seen in the female offspring of as many as 15% of women exposed to DES during pregnancy.
  - uterine hypoplasia.
  - T-shaped uterine cavity.
  - abnormal transverse ridges.
  - stenoses of the cervix.
  - vaginal adenosis.
  - increased risk of vaginal clear cell carcinoma.

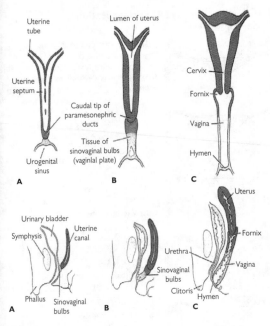

Fig. 1.2 Normal Mullerian development.

American Fertility Society (AFS) classification of Mullerian anomalies

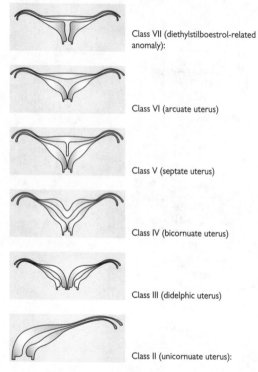

Class VII (diethylstilboestrol-related anomaly):

Class VI (arcuate uterus)

Class V (septate uterus)

Class IV (bicornuate uterus)

Class III (didelphic uterus)

Class II (unicornuate uterus):

Fig. 1.3 American Fertility Society (AFS) classification of Mullerian anomalies.

Hand–foot–genital syndrome

This is a very rare autosomal dominant condition as a result of 7 p15–p14.2 mutations in the **Hox13A** gene. It results in skeletal anomalies in distal limbs and urogenital abnormalities:

- short, proximally placed thumbs with hypoplastic thenar eminences.
- ulnar deviation of the second finger.
- clinodactyly of the fifth finger.
- short, medially deviated halluces.
- brachydactyly of the second to fifth toes.
- shortening of the carpals and tarsals.
- bicornuate uterus.
- vaginal septum.
- ectopic localization of ureteric and urethral orifices.
- vesicoureteric reflux and ureteropelvic obstruction has been observed in females as well as in males. Hypospadias in some affected males.

Incomplete regression of the Wolffian system

Parts of the Wolffian ducts may fail to regress completely in females and present as cysts lateral to the Mullerian ducts. Usually they are incidental findings and most are asymptomatic. The epoophoron and the paraoophoron can be found beside the ovary and the mesosalpinx. Cysts of Gartner's ducts (the lower part of the Wolffian ducts) can occur anywhere from the broad ligament down to the vagina and may present as vulval or vaginal masses. Imaging of the renal tract should be performed whenever abnormalities of the Mullerian system are found.

Further information

Androgen Insensitivity Syndrome Support Group http://www.aissg.org/

Steroid hormones

Introduction

Steroid hormones are synthesized mainly in the gonads (testis and ovary), the adrenals and (during gestation) by the fetoplacental unit. They act on both peripheral target tissues and the central nervous system (CNS). Gonadal steroids influence the sexual differentiation of the genitalia and of the brain, determine 2° sexual characteristics during development and sexual maturation, contribute to the maintenance of their functional state in adulthood and control or modulate sexual behaviour. There are five major classes of steroid hormones. They are the progestagens (progestational hormones), glucocorticoids (anti-stressing hormones), mineralocorticoids (Na+ uptake regulators), androgens (male sex hormones) and oestrogens (female sex hormones).

Steroids are lipophilic, low molecular weight compounds derived from cholesterol which contains a ring system (cyclopentanophenanthrene ring) which is not broken down in mammalian cells. Cholesterol (Fig. 2.1) contains 27 carbons, all of which are derived from acetate. Cholesterol, and each of the steroid hormones, has four rings designated A, B, C and D. In steroid hormones, these rings are fused in a *trans* orientation to form an overall planar structure (unlike bile acids where they are in a *cis* formation leading to a curved structure). The conversion of C27 cholesterol to the 18-, 19- and 21-carbon steroid hormones involves the rate-limiting, irreversible cleavage of a 6-carbon residue from cholesterol, producing pregnenolone (C21) plus isocaproaldehyde.

Steroids are extensively metabolized peripherally, notably in the liver, and in their target tissues, where conversion to an active form is sometimes required before they can elicit their biological responses. Steroid metabolism is therefore important not only for the production of these hormones, but also for the regulation of their cellular and physiological actions.

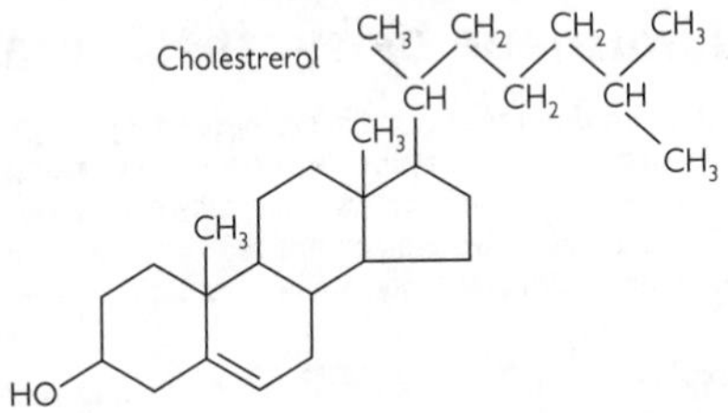

Fig. 2.1 Cholesterol.

Steroid hormone biosynthesis reactions

The particular steroid hormone class synthesized by a given cell type depends upon its complement of peptide hormone receptors, its response to peptide hormone stimulation and its genetically expressed complement of enzymes. Table 2.1 indicates which peptide hormone is responsible for stimulating the synthesis of which steroid hormone.

Table 2.1 Peptide hormones and associated steroid hormones

Peptide hormone	Steroid hormone
Luteinizing hormone (LH)	Progesterone and testosterone
Adrenocorticotrophic hormone (ACTH)	Cortisol
Follicle-stimulating hormone (FSH)	Estradiol
Angiotensin II/III	Aldosterone

The first reaction in converting cholesterol to C18, C19 and C21 steroids involves the cleavage of a 6-carbon group from cholesterol and is the principal committing, regulated and rate-limiting step in steroid biosynthesis. The enzyme system that catalyses the cleavage reaction is known as P450-linked side chain-cleaving enzyme (P450ssc), or desmolase, and is found in the mitochondria of steroid-producing cells, but not in significant quantities in other cells.

Steroids of the adrenal cortex

The adrenal cortex is responsible for production of three major classes of steroid hormones: glucocorticoids, which regulate carbohydrate metabolism; mineralocorticoids, which regulate the body levels of sodium and potassium; and androgens, whose actions are similar to those of steroids produced by the male gonads (see figure 2.2). Adrenal insufficiency is known as Addison disease, and in the absence of steroid hormone replacement therapy can rapidly cause death (in 1–2 weeks). The adrenal cortex is composed of three main tissue regions: zona glomerulosa; zona fasciculata; and zona reticularis. Although the pathway to pregnenolone synthesis is the same in all zones of the cortex, the zones are histologically and enzymatically distinct, with the exact steroid hormone product dependent on the enzymes present in the cells of each zone.

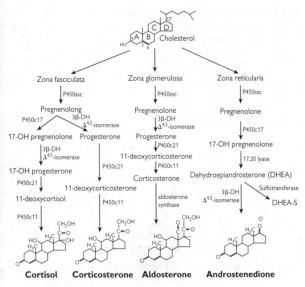

Fig. 2.2 Synthesis of the various adrenal steroid hormones from cholesterol.

Regulation of adrenal steroid synthesis

Adrenocorticotrophic hormone (ACTH) of the hypothalamus regulates the hormone production of the zona fasciculata and zona reticularis (see figure 2.3). ACTH receptors in the plasma membrane activate adenylate cyclase with production of the second messenger, cAMP. The effect of ACTH on the production of cortisol is particularly important, with the result that a classic feedback loop is prominent in regulating the circulating levels of corticotrophin-releasing hormone (CRH), ACTH and cortisol.

Mineralocorticoid secretion from the zona glomerulosa is stimulated by an entirely different mechanism. Angiotensins II and III, derived from the action of the kidney protease renin on liver-derived angiotensinogen, stimulate zona glomerulosa cells by binding a plasma membrane receptor coupled to phospholipase C. Thus, angiotensin II and III binding to their receptor leads to the activation of protein kinase C (PKC) and elevated intracellular Ca^{2+} levels. These events lead to increased P450ssc activity and increased production of aldosterone. In the kidney, aldosterone regulates sodium retention by stimulating gene expression of mRNA for the Na^+/K^+-ATPase responsible for the reaccumulation of sodium from the urine. The interplay between renin from the kidney and plasma angiotensinogen is important in regulating plasma aldosterone levels, sodium and potassium levels, and ultimately blood pressure.

Disorders resulting from defects in steroid biosynthesis

A number of endocrine disorders can be attributed to specific enzyme defects. Thus, inability to secrete normal levels of adrenal steroids may result in congenital adrenal hyperplasia (CAH) following hyperstimulation by ACTH (the negative steroid feedback controlling adrenal activity being lost). In the majority of cases, this syndrome is due to 21-hydroxylase deficiency, and is associated with increased adrenal androgen secretion and partial virilization in girls. Less common adrenal enzyme deficiencies involving either 17-hydroxylase (with a possible increase in mineralocorticoid levels) or 18-hydroxylase (aldosterone may be deficient with normal levels of cortisol) may occur.

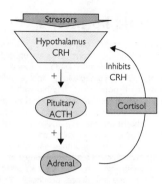

Fig. 2.3 Feedback loop for the control of cortisol production.

Gonadal steroid hormones

The two most important steroids produced by the gonads are testosterone and estradiol (see figure 2.4). These compounds are under tight biosynthetic control, with short and long negative feedback loops that regulate the secretion of FSH and LH by the pituitary, and gonadotropin-releasing hormone (GnRH) by the hypothalamus. The biosynthetic pathway to sex hormones in male and female gonadal tissue includes the production of the androgens—androstenedione and dehydroepiandrosterone. Testes and ovaries contain an additional enzyme, a 17-hydroxysteroid dehydrogenase, that enables androgens to be converted to testosterone. In males, LH binds to Leydig cells, stimulating production of the principal Leydig cell hormone, testosterone. Testosterone is secreted to the plasma and also carried to Sertoli cells by androgen-binding protein (ABP). In Sertoli cells, the Δ-4 double bond of testosterone is reduced, producing dihydrotestosterone (DHT). Testosterone and DHT are carried in the plasma, and delivered to target tissue, by a specific gonadal steroid-binding globulin (GBG). In a number of target tissues, testosterone can be converted to DHT. DHT is the most potent of the male steroid hormones, with an activity that is 10 times that of testosterone. Because of its relatively lower potency, testosterone is sometimes considered to be a prohormone.

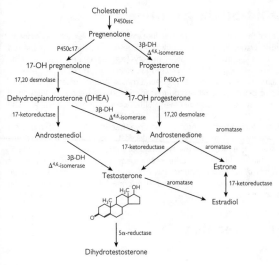

Fig 2.4 Gonadal steroid hormones.

Steroid-binding proteins

Because of their lipophilic properties, free steroid molecules are only sparingly soluble in water. In biological fluids, they are found either in a conjugated form, i.e. linked to a hydrophilic moiety (e.g. as sulfate or glucuronide derivatives), or bound to proteins (non-covalent, reversible binding). In the plasma, unconjugated steroids are found mostly bound to carrier proteins. Binding to plasma albumin, accounting for 20–50% of the bound fraction, is rather unspecific, whereas binding to either corticosteroid-binding globulin (CBG) or the sex hormone-binding globulin (SHBG) is based on more stringent stereospecific criteria. The free fraction (1–10% of the total plasma concentration) is usually considered to represent the biologically active fraction. Apart from the two functions mentioned above, the major roles of plasma binding proteins seem to be (1) to act as a 'buffer' or reservoir for active hormones and (2) to protect the hormone from peripheral metabolism (notably by liver enzymes) and increase the half-life of biologically active forms.

Further reading

Griffin JE, Ojeda SR, ed. *Textbook of Endocrine Physiology*, 5th edn. Oxford: Oxford University Press, 2004.

Menarche and adolescent gynaecology

Introduction

Puberty marks the change from childhood to adolescence, with in girls the development of breasts and 2° sexual hair and with the onset of menstruation. At the same time there is a period of accelerated growth. The age at which the changes take place is variable, but it is abnormal for there to be no signs of 2° sexual development at the age of 14yrs.

The trigger for the changes to start is an increasing frequency and amplitude of gonadotrophin release. The ovaries are then stimulated to produce oestrogen which acts on the breast tissue to promote growth. This usually begins at around the age of 9 and takes about 5yrs to be complete. Pubic hair is stimulated by the release of androgens from the ovaries and the adrenal glands.

The age of menarche in girls appears to be decreasing, particularly in African-American girls. Factors such as general health, nutrition (weight) and exercise all seem to have a role in the age of onset.

Hypothalamic–pituitary–gonadal axis

During fetal life, GnRH activity from the hypothalamus (which is present from ~20 weeks) is suppressed by the steroid production from the feto-placental unit. The ovaries therefore have minimal oestrogen output. During infancy there is an increase in GnRH activity in boys aged 6 months and girls aged ~12 months. This leads to an increase in production of testosterone in boys and oestradiol in girls. At this early age, the feedback mechanism to the pituitary is immature. As this feedback mechanism matures over a few months in childhood, the FSH and LH levels decrease. In girls, this leads to the lowest levels of FSH and LH at ~4yrs old.

At ~6yrs of age in girls there is an increase in the amplitude and frequency of GnRH production from the hypothalamus. This is then associated with the onset of diurnal rhythms of FSH, LH and steroids (see figure 3.1). Puberty progresses with an increase in nocturnal amplitude of LH and a gradual change to the adult pattern of 90min pulses. This is similar in boys and girls.

Boys. In boys, this diurnal rhythm results in peak testosterone in the early morning leading to erections; boys enter puberty ~6 months later than girls but are fertile earlier, with spermaturia from 6mL of testicular volume.

Girls. In girls, the diurnal rhythm results in a rise in oestrogens later in the night as it requires aromatization, thus giving peak values mid-morning. Subsequent ovulatory cycles develop ~2yrs after menarche.

FSH pulsatility shows no diurnal variation at any stage, with only a slight increase in amplitude but not frequency as puberty progresses.

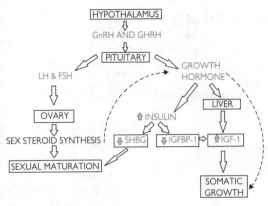

Fig. 3.1 The origins, target organs and fedback mechanisms providing the hyphothalamic–Pituitary–Gonadal axis.

Stages of puberty

In girls, breast and pubic hair development is described in five stages following the classification by Marshall and Tanner (see figure 3.2).

- Sexual characteristics appear in 95% of girls between 8.5 and 13yrs.
- Breast development occurs between 10 and 12.5yrs (average age breast stage II = 11.2yrs).
- Pubic hair usually occurs 6 months after breasts start, although before breasts in one-third.
- 1yr later, adolescent growth spurt.
- Menarche: 12–15yrs, as growth spurt wanes, average age 13yrs.

Marshall and Tanner staging

Stage	Breast	Pubic hair
I	Pre-adolescent, elevation of papilla only	No pubic hair
II	Breast bud—elevation of breast papilla as small mound; enlargement of areolar diameter	Sparse growth of long downy hair along labia
III	Further enlargement but no separation of contours	Hair coarser, darker and more curled; over mons
IV	Projection of areola and papilla to form 2° mound above the level of breast	Adult-type hair but no spread to thigh
V	Mature, areola recessed to general contour of breast	Adult, with horizontal upper border and spread to thigh

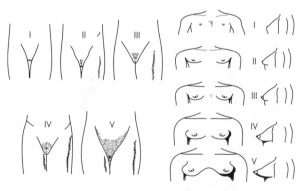

Fig 3.2 Marshall and Tanner stages of puberty.

Precocious puberty

Precocious onset of puberty is defined as occurring younger than 2 SD before the average age; <8yrs old in females and <9yrs in males. Its incidence is ~1 per 5000–10 000 individuals.

Causes of precious puberty

- Idiopathic: family history, overweight/obese accounts for 74% girls (60% boys). Transforming growth factor (TGF)-α may stimulate GnRH secretion.
- McCune–Albright syndrome (café au lait spots and polyostotic fibrous dysplasia).
- Tumours of the adrenal or ovary producing steroids, Peutz–Jeghers syndrome.
- Cerebral tumours: intra-cranial lesions (tumours, hydrocephalus, CNS malformations, irradiation, trauma)—suspect tumour if <3yrs old.
- Ingestion of exogenous oestrogens.

The management of precocious puberty is initially to investigate and exclude tumours. A GnRH agonist (depot) can used for suppression of the hypothalamic–pituitary–gonadal axis. It is important to assess bone age (wrist) to predict potential epiphyseal fusion, and they may benefit from giving growth hormone, but this will depend on the age.

Delayed puberty

Delayed onset of puberty is defined as occurring older than 2 SD after the average age; >13.4yrs old in females >14yrs in males.

A detailed history should be taken asking about general health. In girls, the age at which breast and pubic hair development started and if the girl had a growth spurt or still appears to be growing. Any chronic illness may lead to constitutional delay in puberty. Examination should include accurate measurement of height and, in the female case, breast and pubic hair development. An internal examination should not be performed on girls.

Investigations

- Measurement of gonadotrophins—FSH and LH—and oestrogen.
- Karotyping.
- Ultrasound scan of the pelvis to confirm the presence of uterus and ovaries.
- Possibly X-ray to determine bone age.

Causes of delayed puberty

General

- Constitutional delay of growth and puberty. This is the most common condition seen by paediatric endocrinologists. It is usually associated with a positive family history, short stature, delayed epiphyseal maturation and relatively short upper body. The height prognosis may be appropriate for parental centiles, although in severe cases the upper body may remain short. Treatment may be for psychological reasons, with low dose ethinylestradiol (EE). Usually with the onset of breast development and a growth spurt, the problem resolves.
- Malabsorption (e.g. coeliac disease, inflammatory bowel disease).
- Underweight (dieting/anorexia nervosa, overexercise).
- Other chronic disease (malignancy, asthma, β-thalassaemia major).

Gonadal failure (hypergonadotrophic hypogonadism)

- Turner's syndrome (see Chapter 1).
- Postmalignancy (chemotherapy, local radiotherapy or surgical removal).
- Polyglandular autoimmune syndromes.

Gonadotrophin deficiency

- Congenital hypogonadotrophic hypogonadism (± anosmia). There are a number of possible diagnoses in this category:
  - idiopathic
  - Kallmann's syndrome (X-linked):
    - — impaired migration of GnRH neurons
    - — anosmia, disturbance of colour vision, dyskinesis
  - Prader–Willi syndrome (autosomal dominant, chromosome 15): obesity, muscle hypotonia, mental retardation, short stature, small hands/feet, cryptorchidism
  - mutations in the pathway for GnRH secretion and action (KAL, DAX1, GnRH receptor, etc.).

These cases of hypogonadotrophic hypogonadism may be difficult to distinguish from constitutional delay. Sometimes a GnRH test can be helpful, but results may be unreliable.

- Hypothalamic/pituitary lesions (tumours, post-radiotherapy). Rare inactivating mutations of genes encoding LH, FSH or their receptors.

The management of delay in puberty will follow the diagnosis, but is usually low dose oestradiol (2mcg slowly rising) or pulsatile GnRH or gonadotrophin (FSH + LH) therapy.

Further reading

Lissaue T, Clayde G. *Illustrated Textbook of Paediatrics*, 2nd revised edn. Mosby, 2001.

Ovaries and the menstrual cycle

Introduction

Normally, ovulation occurs once a month in the fertile age range between menarche and menopause, although anovulation generally occurs at the extremes of reproductive life. A cycle is regarded as normal if the duration is 24–35 days. The time between menstruation and ovulation is termed the follicular phase and between ovulation and the next menstruation, the luteal phase. Ovulation itself is the release of a mature, fertilizable oocyte from the dominant follicle, the culmination of an integrated, synchronized interplay of hormones from three principle sources:

- Anterior hypothalamus.
  - gonadotrophin-releasing hormone (GnRH).
- Anterior pituitary.
  - follicle-stimulating hormone (FSH).
  - luteinizing hormone (LH).
- Ovaries.
  - 17-β estradiol.
  - progesterone.

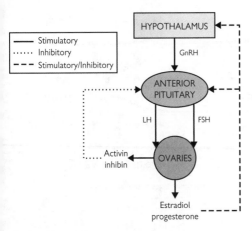

Fig. 4.1 The origins, target organs and feedback mechanisms involving the hypothalamic–pituitary–ovarian axis H = hyphothalamus, P = pituitary, O = ovary and U = Uterus.

In addition, fine tuning is provided by inhibin, activin, follistatin and various growth factors.

Ovulation is achieved through the synchronization of the timing of release and quantity of the various hormones involved, which change throughout the cycle as a result of feedback mechanisms. Fig. 4.1 is a very simple representation of the origin, target organ and feedback mechanisms involving the hypothalamic–pituitary–ovarian axis, and Fig. 4.2 is a diagrammatic representation of the important hormone levels at different stages in the cycle.

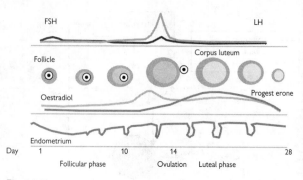

Fig. 4.2 Hormone levels at various stages of the ovulatory cycle.

Hormones

GnRH

GnRH is secreted in a pulsatile fashion from nerve endings in the hypothalamus into the portal vessels running a short course to the anterior pituitary where it induces the synthesis and release of FSH and LH. GnRH is undetectable in the peripheral circulation, but its pulsatile release, about once every hour, can be estimated from the LH pulses. Both the frequency and amplitude of GnRH pulses vary greatly throughout the ovulatory cycle and are much less frequent but of greater amplitude in the luteal phase compared with the follicular phase. The pattern of GnRH release is influenced by feedback mechanisms on the hypothalamus and dictate the pattern of release of FSH and LH.

FSH

Immediately preceding menstruation FSH levels start to rise as corpus luteum function fades, and they reach a peak around day 3 of menstruation. The FSH-stimulated growth of antral follicles, granulosa cell proliferation and differentiation, and aromatase action produce rising concentrations of estradiol and inhibin B which exert a negative feedback mechanism. Other than a temporary increase at the time of the mid-cycle LH surge, FSH remains low until the end of the luteal phase.

FSH has several roles. It promotes:
• Granulosa cell proliferation and differentiation.
• Antral follicle development.
• Oestrogen production.
• Induction of LH receptors on the dominant follicle.
• Inhibin synthesis.

LH

LH is the main promotor of the constant production of androgens, the substrate of ovarian steroid hormones, from theca cells. Concentrations of LH are uneventfully low throughout the ovulatory cycle, except for one tumultuous rise at mid-cycle to 10–20 times the resting levels. This surge lasts for 36–48h and is brought about by a dramatic effect of rapidly rising estradiol levels which reach a certain concentration and initiate a switch from negative to positive feedback.

The preovulatory surge has several functions:
• Triggering of ovulation and follicular rupture.
• Disruption of the cumulus–oocyte complex.
• Induction of the resumption of oocyte meiotic maturation.
• Luteinization of granulosa cells.

Estradiol

17-β estradiol, the most important oestrogen, is produced by granulosa cells under the influence of FSH, which promotes the action of the enzyme aromatase in converting basic androgens to oestrogen. The key functions of estradiol are:
• Endometrial development.
• Triggering of the LH surge at mid-cycle.

- Suppression of FSH concentrations so aiding in the selection of the dominant follicle and preventing multifollicular development in the mid- to late follicular phase.

Estradiol concentrations rise rapidly following menstruation to reach a peak in the late follicular phase and induce the LH surge. A slight decrease following ovulation is revived by production from the corpus luteum, until dropping sharply immediately before menstruation.

Progesterone

The main function of progesterone is to stimulate a secretory endometrium containing multiple tortuous glands receptive to a fertilized embryo, allowing it to implant. It also stimulates the expression of genes needed for implantation.

As progesterone is produced by luteinized granulosa cells, its concentration only rises to significant amounts following ovulation and declines rapidly with the demise of the corpus luteum before menstruation. Progesterone reaches peak levels in the mid-luteal phase. A blood sample for progesterone at this time, e.g. day 21 of a 28-day cycle or day 28 of a 35-day cycle, is used to confirm ovulation.

The ovary

During the reproductive life span, the ovary is a very dramatically changing organ. Fig. 4.3 is a diagrammatic representation of ovarian morphology. The inner, medullary or stromal, section is made up of connective tissue inundated with small capillaries and adrenergic nerves. The cortex contains an enormous number of oocyte-containing follicles ranging from ~300 000 at menarche to 1500 at menopause. There is a constant state of flux in the various stages of development of the follicles from primordial (an oocyte with a single layer of granulosa cells around it), through 1° and 2° stages with increasing numbers of layers of granulosa cells, the antral stage containing follicular fluid, to a fully fledged, preovulatory follicle. A corpus luteum can be seen in the luteal phase of the cycle, and the picture is completed by the presence of corpora albicans (remnants of degenerate corpora lutea).

Although much of this changing picture of stages of follicular development is dependent on the stage of the (gonadotrophin-dependent) ovulatory cycle, there is a constant, non-FSH-dependent, progression in development of primordial to potentially ovulatory follicles being available at the start of the ovulatory cycle, a process that may take ~10 weeks.

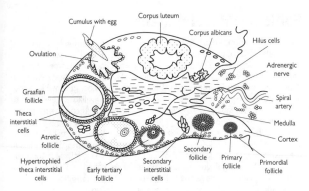

Fig. 4.3 Diagrammatic representation of ovarian morphology.

Follicular development

One follicle a month (i.e. ~400 in a reproductive life span) will be selected to ovulate. The remainder, 99.9% of those that started life in the ovary, become atretic. The earliest stage of follicular selection starts some 10 weeks before the cycle for which it is intended. This is a constant non-FSH-dependent step-up from primordial to several surviving, potentially ovulatory follicles 2–5mm in diameter, which are made available. Sensitivity to FSH then comes into play to select the follicle for further growth, granulosa cell differentiation and multiplication. As oestrogen and inhibin are produced by growing follicles, FSH concentrations are decreased, making it less available. The follicle most sensitive to FSH becomes dominant and the rest fade into atresia, starved of FSH. The dominant follicle is the main producer of estradiol due to aromatase action stimulated by FSH. The dominant follicle also develops LH receptors in the late follicular phase in preparation for the LH surge and impending ovulation.

Causes of anovulation and oligo-ovulation

The causes of anovulation and oligo-ovulation (<9 ovulations in 1yr) are listed according to a modified World Health Organization (WHO) classification. The advantage of this type of classification is that it is treatment orientated, i.e. once the cause of the anovulation has been determined, the starting treatment for the induction of ovulation in that particular condition will be indicated. The four groups of causes are:

- Hypothalamic–pituitary failure (WHO Group I).
- Hypothalamic–pituitary dysfunction (WHO Group II).
- Ovarian failure (WHO Group III).
- Hyperprolactinaemia (WHO Group IV).

Hypothalamic–pituitary failure

Otherwise known as hypogonadotrophic hypogonadism, this is a condition in which gonadotrophin concentrations are so low as to be unable to stimulate follicle development or ovarian steroidogenesis. Anovulation and amenorrhoea are the consequences. There are several possible causes of this condition:

- Weight-related amenorrhoea—the most common hypothalamic cause of anovulation, due to loss of weight as a result of severe dieting or frank anorexia nervosa.
- Exercise-related amenorrhoea—caused by very strenuous exercise such as marathon running and other athletic pursuits, and not uncommon in ballet dancers.
- Stress-related—even moderate stress, e.g. moving house, before examinations, long journeys involving time shifts, etc.
- Kallmann's syndrome—hypothalamic amenorrhoea associated with anosmia (loss of the sense of smell).
- Debilitating diseases.
- Craniopharyngioma.
- Idiopathic—probably the most common 'cause' of 1° amenorrhoea.
- Surgical—hypophysectomy.
- Radiotherapy for tumours of the pituitary or surrounding area.
- Sheehan's syndrome—hypogonadotrophic hypogonadism and hypopituitarism following severe postpartum haemorrhage.

Hypothalamic–pituitary dysfunction

Characterized by normal FSH and estradiol concentrations, usually presenting as oligo- or amenorrhoea and comprising ~90% of all ovulatory disorders. In this group of ovulatory disorders, the vast majority are associated with polycystic ovary syndrome (PCOS).

About 75% of all ovulatory disorders causing infertility are due to PCOS and are characterized by clinical and/or biochemical hyperandrogenism (hirsutism, persistent acne, raised testosterone concentrations) and a typical polycystic appearance of the ovary on ultrasound examination. Many women with PCOS are overweight or obese and hyperinsulinaemic. The basic aetiology is unknown but it is thought to be associated with an overproduction of androgens by the ovaries which, in the majority of these women, seems to be genetic in origin. For a full description of this syndrome, see Chapter 5.

Ovarian failure

Ovarian failure is characterized by amenorrhoea, hypo-oestrogenism and high concentrations of FSH (often >25IU/L). It is often accompanied at its onset by hot flushes. The ovaries in this condition are unable to respond to endogenous or exogenous FSH as they are either completely devoid of oocytes or have a severely depleted reserve of oocytes. Possible causes are:

- The onset of a 'natural' menopause (>40 years of age).
- Premature menopause (<40 years of age)—which may be familial, or caused by a systemic autoimmune abnormality, chemotherapy or direct radiation of the ovaries, but the underlying cause is often idiopathic.
- Chromosomal abnormalities, e.g. Turner's syndrome (45, XO) characterized by its typical physical features of short stature, cubitus valgus, webbed neck and 'streak' ovaries, and sometimes associated with aortic stenosis, presenting with 1° amenorrhoea.

Hyperprolactinaemia

The presenting features of this cause of oligo- or anovulation are oligo/amenorrhoea, infertility and often, but not always, galactorrhoea. Anovulation due to hyperprolactinaemia is usually associated with serum prolactin concentrations, measured at least 2h after awakening, more than twice the upper limit of normal. Mildly raised concentrations of prolactin may be found in conditions such as PCOS and mild, transient stress, but in these cases are not a 1° cause of anovulation and do not require specific treatment.

The major causes of hyperprolactinaemia associated with anovulation are:

- Pituitary adenoma (prolactinoma)—almost invariably benign tumours that secrete prolactin. According to their size they may be termed macroadenomas (>10mm in diameter) or microadenomas (<10mm) when visualized by MRI or CT scan. When large, these adenomata may impinge on the optic chiasma inducing a bitemporal hemianopia.
- Hypothyroidism. Thyroid-stimulating hormone (TSH) is released from the hypothalamus by TSH-releasing hormone, which is thought to be a prolactin-releasing hormone. As TSH concentrations (and, by inference, those of TSH-releasing hormone) are often elevated in hypothyroid conditions, these may often be associated with hyperprolactinaemia sufficient to cause anovulation.
- Medications—many drugs used in psychiatric conditions, as sedatives or anti-emetics, suppress the hypothalamic secretion of dopamine. As dopamine is thought to be a prolactin-inhibiting factor, these medications can often induce hyperprolactinaemia and a consequent anovulation. Oral contraceptives and other oestrogen-containing medications may also induce a mild hyperprolactinaemia, often associated with galactorrhoea.

The treatment of these causes of anovulation is dealt with in Chapter 14.

Polycystic ovary syndrome

Introduction

In 1935 Stein and Leventhal first described the polycystic ovary as a frequent cause of irregular ovulation or anovulation in obese women seeking treatment for subfertility. The initial management of the condition was surgical, with wedge resection of the ovaries resulting in restoration of ovulation in the majority of cases. In the last two decades, the polycystic ovary syndrome (PCOS) has been studied intensely and, although the exact aetiology still escapes us, considerable knowledge of the prevalence, pathophysiology and management of the syndrome has been gained.

Aetiology

Uncertainty still surrounds the exact aetiology of PCOS, although there is increasing evidence for genetic factors. The syndrome clusters in families, and prevalence rates in first-degree relatives are 5–6 times higher than in the general population. About 70% of cases appear to be genetically transmitted. Intra-uterine exposure of the female fetus to an excess of androgens is an aetiologogical hypothesis finding increasing favour, although the source of the excess androgens is unknown. The syndrome may also be acquired by an exposure to excess androgens at any time during the fertile time of life.

Pathophysiology

PCOS is a very heterogeneous syndrome as regards both clinical presentation and laboratory manifestations. While the basic dysfunction seems to lie within the ovary, the clinical expression and severity of the symptoms are dependent on extra-ovarian factors such as obesity, insulin resistance and LH concentrations.

There are four main disturbances which may be involved in the pathophysiology of the syndrome:

- Abnormal ovarian morphology: ~6–8 times more preantral and small antral follicles are present in the polycystic ovary compared with the normal ovary. They arrest in development at a size of 2–9mm, have a slow rate of atresia and are sensitive to exogenous FSH stimulation. An enlarged stromal volume is invariably present, and a total ovarian volume >10mL is often witnessed.
- Excessive ovarian androgen production lies at the heart of the syndrome. Almost every enzymatic action within the polycystic ovary which encourages androgen production is accelerated. Both insulin and LH, alone and in combination, exacerbate androgen production (Fig. 5.1).
- Hyperinsulinaemia due to insulin resistance occurs in ~80% of women with PCOS and central obesity, but also in ~30–40% of lean women with PCOS. This is thought to be due to a postreceptor defect affecting glucose transport, and is unique to women with PCOS. Insulin resistance, significantly exacerbated by obesity, is a key factor in the pathogenesis of anovulation and hyperandrogenism (Fig. 5.2).
- An abnormality of pancreatic β-cell function has also been described.
- Excessive serum concentrations of LH are detected on single spot blood samples in ~40–50% of women with PCOS. High LH concentrations are more commonly found in lean rather than obese women. Although FSH serum concentrations are often within the low normal range, an intrinsic inhibition of FSH action may be present. Prolactin concentrations may be slightly elevated.

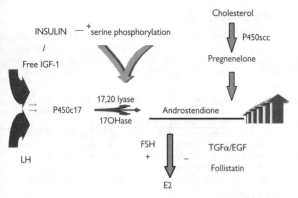

Fig. 5.1 Mechanisms of excessive androgen production in the polycystic ovary.

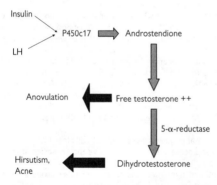

Fig. 5.2 Insulin action as a key factor in the pathogenesis of anovulation and hyperandrogenism.

Management

The management of PCOS depends on the presenting symptoms. Whether these are symptoms of hyperandrogenism such as hirsutism and acne, oligo- or amenorrhoea, or anovulatory infertility, the first-line treatment for the overweight or frankly obese must be loss of weight.

Weight loss

Obesity is a common feature in the majority of women with PCOS. Increased truncal–abdominal fat in women with PCOS exacerbates insulin resistance and hyperandrogenism, and, consequently, the severity of the symptoms. Fortunately, the reverse is also true in that diet and exercise ('lifestyle changes') are effective treatment. The loss of just 5% or more of body weight is capable of considerably reducing the severity of hirsutism and acne and restoring menstrual regularity and ovulation. A motivation-inducing explanation of these facts should be given at the first consultation.

Hirsutism and acne

As many as 92% of women with hirsutism and 84% with persistent acne have PCOS as the underlying cause. A full description of management can be found in Chapter 6.

- The first step for those who are overweight should be lifestyle changes to induce loss of weight. A loss of 5–10% of body weight is enough to greatly improve hirsutism within 6 months of weight reduction in the majority of women.
- The combination of an anti-androgen, cyproterone acetate (CPA, 2mg/day), and ethinylestradiol (EE, 35 micrograms/day) (co-cyprindiol) is very effective treatment when given cyclically. A significant improvement of acne can be achieved after 3 months and of hirsutism after 9 months of treatment. The addition of CPA in a dose of 10–100mg/day on the first 10 days of the combined medication has proved effective for more severe cases.
- Combined oral contraceptives (COCs) will also slowly improve hirsutism and acne, but are less effective than specific anti-androgen medications.
- Other anti-androgen medications used include spironolactone, flutamide and finasteride. These are mostly used in the USA where CPA is unavailable. Contraception is needed during their use.
- Mechanical means of hair removal and more traditional treatment for persistent acne may also be used, especially when waiting for medication to take effect.
- Metformin, a well-established anti-diabetic agent, is capable of reducing the degree of hirsutism but is not usually recommended as first-line treatment when hirsutism is the main presenting symptom.

Anovulation and infertility

- Weight loss—should be the first-line treatment for the overweight desiring pregnancy. A reduction of 5% or more of body weight is often enough to restore ovulation and induce pregnancy, and is also important for reducing miscarriage rates.

- Clomifene citrate—the first-line medication for the induction of ovulation. Given in a dose of 50–100mg/day from day 4 to 8 of a spontaneous or progestin-induced menstruation, clomifene will restore ovulation in ~75% and induce pregnancy in ~35–40%. Failure to induce ovulation is more common in the very obese and those with very high serum androgen, insulin or LH concentrations. Failure to respond to 150mg/day, an endometrial thickness of <7mm at mid-cycle or failure to conceive following six ovulatory cycles require a change of treatment mode. (For a detailed account, see Chapter 14).
- Metformin, a well-established oral anti-diabetic agent, is capable of increasing ovulatory frequency in women with PCOS, apparently by decreasing insulin and androgen concentrations, in a dose of 1500–2500mg/day (unlicensed). Its efficacy does not seem to depend on the presence of demonstrable insulin resistance, there is no evidence of teratogenicity and it does not induce hypoglycaemia in women with euglycaemia. Although clomifene is more efficient in inducing ovulation and pregnancy as first-line treament as a mono-agent, metformin in combination with clomifene or added to clomifene for women who have proved clomifene resistant is a worthwhile strategy before having to proceed to gonadotrophin treatment. Gastrointestinal side-effects are not uncommon.
- Low-dose gonadotrophin therapy—designed to induce ovulation and conception while minimizing the complications due to multifollicular development, ovarian hyperstimulation syndrome (OHSS) and multiple pregnancies. Using a starting dose of 50–75IU/day of FSH or human menopausal gonadotrophin (hMG) without a change of dose for the first 7–14 days and only small incremental dose rises of 25–37.5IU for a minimum of 7 days where necessary, pregnancy rates of >20% per cycle may be expected while OHSS is almost completely eliminated and multiple pregnancy rates are <6%. hCG should be withheld if >3 follicles of diameter >16mm are induced. Fuller details can be found in Chapter 14.
- Laparoscopic ovarian drilling (LOD) using cautery or laser has proved effective in restoring ovulation and inducing pregnancy, particularly in women of normal weight and with high concentrations of LH. Multiple pregnancy rate is low. Some units employ LOD when clomifene resistance is apparent; most others following failure of gonadotrophin therapy.
- IVF can be successfully employed for anovulatory women with PCOS when a further infertility-causing factor is involved or when the above methods of ovulation induction have been unsuccessful.

A suggested algorithm for the induction of ovulation for women with PCOS is shown in Fig. 5.3.

For a more detailed account of these methods of ovulation induction, see Chapter 14.

Long-term health implications of PCOS

- Women with PCOS who are obese, hyperinsulinaemic and hyperandrogenic are at substantial risk for the development of metabolic syndrome (syndrome X). If they remain untreated, the risk of developing diabetes mellitus is 7 times greater and hypertension 4 times greater than in the general population. Both these conditions, and dyslipidaemia and hyperhomocysteinaemia, also common in PCOS, increase the risk of cardio- and cerebrovascular disease. Weight loss, diet and exercise can reduce these dangers.
- Women with PCOS have an increased incidence of gestational diabetes and of pregnancy-induced hypertension.
- Endometrial cancer has a 5-fold increased incidence in PCOS due to unopposed oestrogen action on the endometrium. This may be prevented by treating with a progestin-containing medication used cyclically or once every 3 months to induce uterine bleeding. Endometrial hyperplasia may be treated similarly.

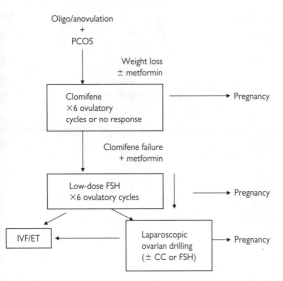

Fig. 5.3 A suggested algorithm for the induction of ovulation for women with PCOS. Although less efficient than clomifene as first-line treatment, metformin is also capable of inducing ovulation. Laparoscopic ovarian drilling may be applied at any stage after clomifene resistance is evident.

Further reading

Balen A, Conway GS, Homburg R, Legro R. *Polycystic Ovary Syndrome—A Guide to Clinical Management.* London and New York: Taylor & Francis, 2005.

Hirsutism and virilization

Introduction

- Hirsutism in the female is an excess of pigmented, thick terminal hair that appears in a male distribution in androgen-sensitive areas. These areas include face, chest, abdomen and thighs. An excess of androgens will produce such hair growth in a male distribution.
- Virilization is a much more progressive and serious form of hyperandrogenism and may include, in addition to hirsutism, male-pattern baldness, cliteromegaly, muscle development and deepening of the voice.
- Hirsutism may be due to hyperandrogenism from ovarian, adrenal or iatrogenic (drug) sources. If not associated with irregular menstruation, it is probably familial, without underlying pathology.
- Ethnic differences exist in the symptom of hirsutism, e.g. Mediterranean and Indian ethnicities may typically have more facial and body hair than do South and East Asian and North European communities.

Pathophysiology

Androgens stimulate the development of the pilosebaceous unit, a common skin structure that gives rise to both hair follicles and sebaceous glands, found throughout the body except on the palms, soles and lips.

Before puberty, body hair is primarily composed of fine, short, unpigmented vellous hairs which during pubarche are stimulated by androgens to become coarse, pigmented, thickened terminal hairs.

Following puberty in the female, excessive exposure to androgens may cause hirsutism by overstimulation of the transformation of fine, unpigmented vellous hairs to coarse, pigmented thickened terminal hairs in skin areas sensitive to the effects of androgens. However, paradoxically, scalp hair responds to severe prolonged hyperandrogenism by loss of hair.

The hair growth cycle consists of three phases: active growth, resting phase and shedding. The length of this cycle varies from 4 months on the face to 3 years on the scalp. This is important to know when assessing the response to treatment.

Androgens

- Androgens are the main regulators of terminal hair growth. Testosterone is a strong androgen which binds to intracellular androgen receptors in the skin and is converted by 5α-reductase to dihydrotestosterone (DHT) which has even more potent androgen effects on the hair follicle and sebaceous gland. The concentration of free, biologically active testosterone, a crucial factor, is 2%. Testosterone is bound by sex-hormone binding globulin (SHBG) (65%) and albumin (33%). Testosterone itself, obesity and insulin lower SHBG concentrations, inducing increased activity of androgen action. The androgen receptor content will also influence the degree of androgen action on the hair follicle.
- Androgens are produced by ovaries and adrenal glands. The basic androgen is androstendione produced by both ovaries and adrenals, and this is converted to testosterone, the major androgen, in both these organs. At the level of the skin, testosterone is converted by 5α-reductase to DHT, which has a potent effect on the pilosebaceous unit. Dehydroepiandrosterone and its sulfate (DHEAS) are produced mainly by the adrenals.
- Ovarian androgens originate from theca cells, and their production is regulated by LH and insulin. Adrenal androgen production is regulated by ACTH.
- Hyperandrogenism from ovarian, adrenal or iatrogenic sources may produce symptoms of hirsutism, acne, alopecia or virilism, depending on its degree.

History and examination

The rapidity of the onset and progress of hirsutism is a vital diagnostic pointer.

- A rapid progression of symptoms, especially when accompanied by virilization, may be indicative of an ovarian or adrenal tumour.
- A more insidious onset and progress of symptoms in the late teens when accompanied by oligo- or amenorrhoea is due to polycystic ovary syndrome (PCOS) in ~90% of cases.
- Hirsutism above the upper lip and on the limbs, especially when unaccompanied by menstrual disturbance or polycystic ovaries, is more likely to be familial. Enquiries or examination of other family members should be made.
- On examination, in order to determine a baseline before initiating treatment, a full description of the location and severity of the hirsutism is required. This often suffices clinically, but a more specific estimation may be performed using a modified Ferriman–Gallwey score, the Lorenzo scale of hirsutism (Fig. 6.1).
- Other signs of hyperandrogenism and virilization should be sought, i.e. acne, male-pattern balding or frank alopecia, or enlarged clitoris. Acanthosis nigricans, dark staining of the skin in the axillary or neck regions, indicates insulin resistance and is associated with obesity and PCOS.

Aetiology

- Familial.
- Ovarian.
  - PCOS.
  - Androgen-producing tumours.
- Adrenal.
  - Congenital adrenal hyperplasia (CAH).
  - Cushing's syndrome.
  - Neoplasms.
- Iatrogenic.
  - Anabolic steroids.
  - Danazol.
  - Phenytoin.

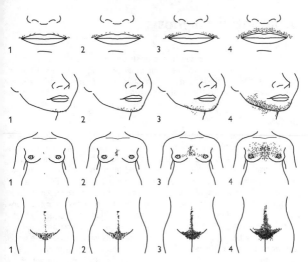

Fig. 6.1 The Lorenzo scale of hirsutism.

Differential diagnosis

Familial

Usually presents as excessive hair growth on the forearms, lower limbs and upper lip, which is often evident in close family members. Ovarian function is normal, periods are regular as are androgen concentrations. Familial hirsutism is both typical and natural in certain populations, such as in some women of Mediterranean ancestry.

PCOS

An insidious onset of hirsutism accompanied by oligo- or amenorrhoea is enough to make the diagnosis of PCOS. In a large majority of cases, this may be confirmed by an ultrasonic vaginal examination of the ovaries demonstrating >12 follicles between 2 and 9mm in diameter and/or an ovarian volume >10mL. Obesity, which often accompanies PCOS, exaggerates the symptoms of hyperandrogenism. Hormonal manifestations are not required for the diagnosis, but raised serum testosterone concentrations are often found. Concentrations of LH are frequently high, especially in women with PCOS of normal weight, and insulin resistance, detected by a fasting glucose:insulin ratio of <4.5, on a glucose tolerance test, or by more sophisticated methods, is very prevalent, especially in the overweight and frankly obese. See Chapter 5 on PCOS for more details.

Androgen-producing tumours

The hallmark of these fortunately rare tumours is a rapid onset and progression of symptoms. Hirsutism may be rapidly followed by symptoms and signs of virilization. Testosterone levels are extremely high, often in the male range with ovarian androgen-producing tumours, and DHEAS levels are very high with adrenal tumours. Ultrasound, MRI or CT scans are required to confirm the diagnosis.

Congenital adrenal hyperplasia (CAH)

CAH is a partial block of enzyme action in the cascade involved in eventual cortisol synthesis in the adrenal. The partial block induces an increased discharge of ACTH and a consequent accumulation of androgens. The most common form is 21-hydroxylase deficiency which is particularly prevalent in Ashkenazi Jews. Almost invariably, the CAH seen by gynaecologists is a mild form of 21-hydroxylase deficiency with an onset of hyperandrogenic symptoms in early adult life (late onset, LOCAH). Very high serum concentrations of 17-hydroxyprogesterone, 10–400 times higher than normal values, establish the diagnosis. Rarer forms of LOCAH, 11β-hydroxylase and 3β-hydroxysteroid dehydrogenase deficiencies, require dynamic testing with ACTH for accurate diagnosis.

PCOS is almost invariably found in association with CAH.

Other possible diagnoses

Luteoma of pregnancy driven by hCG can produce symptoms of hyper-androgenism. They may be diagnosed in the early stages of pregnancy by ultrasound examination, need no treatment and regress spontaneously following delivery. Cushing's syndrome may cause hirsutism but has other very characteristic features which do not usually present to the gynaecologist.

The key laboratory investigations are total testosterone which will be very high (often in the male range) in the case of ovarian androgen-producing tumours, as is DHEAS in adrenal tumours, and these diagnoses must be ruled out especially in the presence of rapidly progressive symptoms. In certain populations, 21-hydroxylase-deficient LOCAH is prevalent and can be excluded by measuring a basal morning serum 17-hydroxyprogesterone concentration (cut-off value, 20nmol/L).

Treatment

- When hirsutism is accompanied by overweight or frank obesity, as is often the case in PCOS, weight loss should be the first line of treatment. For obese women with PCOS, a loss of 5–10% of body weight is enough to improve hirsutism greatly in 40–55% within 6 months of weight reduction. Weight loss has the undoubted advantages of being effective and cheap with no side-effects. Metformin, a well-established oral anti-diabetic agent, is capable of reducing insulin and androgen concentrations in women with PCOS. Although it may have a therapeutic effect on the degree of hirsutism, it cannot be recommended as the first-line treatment when hirsutism is the main presenting symptom.
- Mechanical means of hair removal may be used as a short-term solution to hirsutism or as an adjuvant to medical treatment, especially when waiting for medication to take effect.
- Surgical removal is required for all androgen-producing tumours.
- When LOCAH is the established cause of hirsutism, the administration of dexamethasone, 0.5mg at bedtime, is capable of completely reversing the symptoms. Due to the length of the hair growth cycle, this will take 3–9 months to start the improvement, but no other medication is required.
- Combined oral contraceptives (COCs) that do not contain androgenic progestogen will slowly improve hirsutism by suppressing LH and increasing SHBG concentrations. However, anti-androgenic medications are a more specific and more effective treatment for hirsutism.
- A number of anti-androgen medicines that block the synthesis or action of androgens may be used for the treatment of hirsutism: cyproterone acetate (CPA), spironolactone, flutamide and finasteride.

Excluding North America, a combination of CPA, an orally active progestogen, and ethinylestradiol (EE) is probably the most widely used anti-androgen treatment. CPA has an anti-androgen action at several sites:

- In combination with EE, suppression of LH release by the anterior pituitary.
- Competition for the androgen receptor which it blocks.
- As a progestogen in suppressing the action of 5α-reductase.
- With EE, increases SHBG concentrations.

The combination of CPA (2mg/day) and EE (35 micrograms/day) given cyclically has proved very effective in the treatment of hirsutism and acne, as well as serving as an excellent contraceptive. A reduction of >50% in the hirsutism score has been demonstrated after 9 months of treatment using this minimal dose. The addition of CPA in a dose of 10–100mg/day on the first 10 days of the combined medication has proved effective for more severe cases. Success rates in reversing or severely diminishing symptoms and maintaining improvement with minimal side-effects are high, but patients need to be informed that this treatment is not 'instant' and that at least 3–9 months are needed to see an improvement in hirsutism. The combination of CPA (50mg/day) from days 5 to 10 of the menstrual cycle in combination with EE (35 micrograms/day) successfully arrests the balding process and increases hair regrowth in diffuse androgen-dependent alopecia. This often takes >9 months to achieve, and vitamin B supplements are usually given concurrently. Side-effects of CPA in combination with EE are similar to those of oral contraceptives, are usually mild and transient and include mastodinia, increased appetite, change of libido and headaches. The effects on the lipid profile are usually slight and probably clinically irrelevant, and include an increase in triglycerides and a small increase in cholesterol, mainly due to an increase in the high-density lipoprotein (HDL) fraction.

Spironolactone

Spironolactone is an aldosterone antagonist, widely used in the USA where CPA is unavailable, whose anti-androgen action is exerted by competitive inhibition of testosterone and DHT binding to the androgen receptor. In the usual dose of 100mg/day, spironolactone may induce some menstrual disturbances, particularly polymenorrhoea which is often transient and resolves within a few months, and mild breast tenderness occurs frequently. Spironolactone has been widely used for the treatment of hirsutism, and a 40% reduction of the hirsutism score after 6 months may be expected, similar to that obtained with flutamide and finasteride.

Flutamide

Flutamide is a non-steroidal anti-androgen which has primarily been used in advanced prostatic carcinoma in that it inhibits DHT binding to the androgen receptors. It has also proved effective in the treatment of hirsutism and acne in women. Similar improvements of hirsutism have been reported whether doses of 250 or 500mg/day are used. The efficacy, non-interference with ovulation and generally good tolerance of flutamide have been tempered by rare reports of hepatotoxicity which may be severe, and the incidence of which seems to increase with higher doses. Careful monitoring of liver function is therefore advised if flutamide is to be used for the treatment of hirsutism.

Finasteride

Finasteride acts by inhibiting the activity of 5α-reductase, the enzyme responsible for the conversion of testosterone to DHT, which is particularly potent at hair follicle level. Taken orally in a dose of 1–5mg/day it is effective without any appreciable side-effects, although it may need prolonged treatment to achieve the goal. Finasteride is thought to be effective in the treatment of hirsutism regardless of the cause, as 5α-reductase has a vital role in the androgen regulation of hair growth and its inhibition is thus potentially effective. As with spironolactone and flutamide, contraceptive use is recommended with finasteride in order to avoid the potential risk of feminization of a male fetus.

However effective these anti-androgen medicines may be, they ameliorate symptoms while they are being taken but fail to 'cure' the cause. After the withdrawal of treatment with spironolactone, flutamide or CPA, hirsutism relapses to 60–80% of the original score. The longer the duration of treatment (at least with CPA/EE), the less chance of relapse within a given time. Using long-term treatment with CPA (25–50mg/day) and EE (0.01–0.02mg/day) in a reverse sequential regimen, hirsutism was absent for 6 months in all patients. After 12 months without treatment, 28% had worsened and after 24 months, 44% were still showing an improvement on the original hirsutism score.

An essential element in the successful compliance of the patient on anti-androgen treatment is the accuracy and fullness of information given to her. First and foremost, she should be told that a good clinical response to treatment takes time; secondly, the need for long-term maintenance treatment of 3–4 years, even when obvious clinical improvement has been achieved, and thirdly, the possibility of relapse some time after treatment is terminated.

Amenorrhoea and oligomenorrhoea

Introduction

Amenorrhoea is the absence of menstruation for at least 6 months. 1° amenorrhoea is defined if a menstrual period has never occurred and 2° amenorrhoea after at least one period.

Oligomenorrhoea is the occurrence of menstruation less than once in 35 days to 6 months or <9 times in 1yr.

Aetiology

Physiological amenorrhoea is an acceptable diagnosis:
- Before the onset of menarche, unless this has not occurred before the age of 17yrs.
- Following the menopause, if this occurs after the age of 40yrs.
- During pregnancy.
- During lactation.

All other causes of amenorrhoea and oligomenorrhoea are listed according to a modified World Health Organization (WHO) classification. The five groups of causes are:
- Hypothalamic–pituitary failure (WHO Group I).
- Hypothalamic–pituitary dysfunction (WHO Group II).
- Ovarian failure (WHO Group III).
- Hyperprolactinaemia (WHO Group IV).
- Outflow tract defect (WHO Group V).

The classification of oligo/amenorrhoea, common causes and hormonal profiles are summarized in Table 7.1.

Table 7.1 Classification of oligo/amenorrhoea, common causes and hormonal profiles

WHO Group	Name	Common causes	Hormonal profile
I	Hypothalamic–pituitary failure Hypogonadotrophic Hypogonadism	Weight, exercise, stress related Kallmann's syndrome Sheehan's syndrome Hypophysectomy/ radiotherapy Tumours Idiopathic	Very low FSH, LH, E2
II	Hypothalamic–pituitary dysfunction	PCOS	Low or normal FSH High or normal LH High or normal testosterone
		CAH Cushing's Androgen-producing tumours	High 17-OH prog. High cortisol Very high testosterone
III	Ovarian failure	Autoimmune Infections Surgery/irradiation Gonadal dysgenesis Idiopathic/familial	High FSH, LH (LH may be normal in early stages). Low E2
IV	Hyperprolactinaemia	Pituitary adenoma Medication Stress Hypothyroidism	High prolactin Low FSH, LH High TSH
V	Outflow tract defect	Imperforate hymen Transverse vaginal septum Asherman's syndrome Absent uterus Cervical stenosis Androgen insensitivity Hermaphroditism	Normal Testosterone— male

Hypothalamic–pituitary failure

Amenorrhea in this condition is due to hypogonadotrophic hypogonadism, in which concentrations of both FSH and LH are so low as to be unable to stimulate follicle development or ovarian steroidogenesis. Amenorrhea, anovulation and hypo-oestrogenism are the consequences. There are several possible causes of this condition:

• Weight-related amenorrhoea—a not uncommon cause of amenorrhoea, due to loss of weight during severe dieting or frank anorexia nervosa.
• Exercise-related amenorrhoea—caused by very strenuous exercise such as marathon running and other athletic pursuits, and not uncommon in ballet dancers.
• Stress-related—even moderate stress, e.g. moving house, before examinations, long journeys involving time shifts, etc.
• Kallmann's syndrome—hypothalamic amenorrhoea associated with anosmia (loss of the sense of smell).
• Debilitating systemic diseases.
• Craniopharyngioma.
• Idiopathic—probably the most common 'cause' of 1° amenorrhoea.
• Surgical—hypophysectomy.
• Radiotherapy for tumours of the pituitary or surrounding area.
• Sheehan's syndrome—hypogonadotrophic hypogonadism and hypopituitarism following severe post-partum haemorrhage.

Hypothalamic–pituitary dysfunction

WHO Group II may present as oligo- or amenorrhoea, and comprises the vast majority of these types of disorders that are seen. Characterized by normal FSH and estradiol concentrations, almost all these cases are associated with PCOS. A full description of this syndrome can be found in Chapter 5 but, briefly, PCOS is characterized by oligo- or amenorrhoea, clinical and/or biochemical hyperandrogenism (hirsutism, persistent acne, raised testosterone concentrations) and a typical polycystic appearance of the ovary on ultrasound examination. Two or more of these three diagnostic points are enough to confirm the diagnosis, assuming other causes of hyperandrogenism have been ruled out. Many women with PCOS are overweight or obese, hyperinsulinaemic and infertile. The basic aetiology is unknown, but it is thought to be associated with an overproduction of androgens by the ovaries which, in the majority of these women, seems to be genetic in origin.

Ovarian failure

Ovarian failure is responsible for ~10% of women with 2° amenorrhoea before the age of 40yrs (premature menopause), but may also be a cause of 1° amenorrhoea. This form of amenorrhoea is characterized by hypo-oestrogenism and high concentrations of FSH (often >25IU/L). The ovaries in this condition are unable to respond to endogenous or exogenous FSH as they are either completely devoid of oocytes or have a severely depleted reserve of oocytes. Possible causes are:

Secondary amenorrhea—premature menopause
- Familial/genetic.
- Autoimmune abnormality.
- Iatrogenic—chemotherapy or direct radiation of the ovaries, pelvic surgery.
- Debilitating systemic disease.
- Infectious, e.g. mumps.
- Idiopathic.

Primary amenorrhea
- Chromosomal abnormalities—gonadal dysgenesis, e.g. Turner's syndrome (45, XO) characterized by its typical physical features of short stature, cubitus valgus, webbed neck and 'streak' ovaries, and sometimes associated with aortic stenosis.
- Intersexuality and hermaphroditism.

Hyperprolactinaemia

Hyperprolactinaemia may be a cause of either oligo- or amenorrhoea, infertility and often, but not always, galactorrhoea. (Conversely, galactorrhoea is not always accompanied by hyperprolactinaemia.)

Common causes of hyperprolactinaemia:
- Pituitary adenoma (prolactinoma)—almost invariably benign tumours that secrete prolactin. According to their size they may be termed macroadenomas (>10mm in diameter) or microadenomas (<10mm) when visualized by MRI or CT scan. When large, these adenomata may impinge on the optic chiasma inducing a bi-temporal hemianopia.
- Hypothyroidism. Thyroid-stimulating hormone (TSH)-releasing hormone is also thought to be a prolactin-releasing hormone. As TSH concentrations (and, by inference, TSH-releasing hormone) are often elevated in hypothyroid conditions, these may often be associated with hyperprolactinaemia sufficient to cause oligo- or amenorrhoea.
- Medications—many drugs used in psychiatric conditions, as sedatives or anti-emetics, suppress the hypothalamic secretion of dopamine. As dopamine is thought to be a prolactin-inhibiting factor, these medications can often induce hyperprolactinaemia and a consequent oligo- or amenorrhoea. Oral contraceptives and other oestrogen-containing medications may also induce a mild hyperprolactinaemia, often associated with galactorrhoea.
- Stress, particularly if prolonged, may cause a hyperprolactinaemia sufficient to induce oligo- or amenorrhoea.

Outflow tract defects

Unlike the aforementioned causes of amenorrhea, outflow tract defects are not usually associated with anovulation but with a mechanical defect preventing menstruation.

Possible causes include:
- Imperforate hymen.
- Congenital absence of the uterus (see Chapter 1).
- Transverse vaginal septum.
- Severe intra-uterine adhesions/endometrial damage (Asherman's syndrome).
- Cervical stenosis.

Investigations

The importance of a detailed gynaecological and medical history cannot be emphasized enough. By listening carefully and asking the correct direct questions followed by a thorough gynaecological and general physical examination, the clues obtained will often point toward the diagnosis and dictate the order in which examinations should be performed. Using this approach and good common sense, laboratory examinations, expense and time can be limited to a minimum. A suggested 'check-list' is presented in Table 7.2.

Table 7.2 A suggested check-list for history taking and physical examination of the amenorrhoeic patient

History

Age—female partner
Occupation
Previous pregnancies
Duration of amenorrhea—primary or secondary
Previous regularity of menstruation
Past medical and surgical history
Intercurrent illnesses/medications/drugs/alcohol
Family history
Previous contraception
Age at menarche
Sexual activity/problems
Direct questions where relevant—

    Sense of smell? Abdominal pain? Physical activity?
    Serious changes in weight/diet?
    Hot flushes? Hirsutism, acne, galactorrhoea?

Examination

Body build
Weight, height, body mass index
General physical examination
Distribution of hair growth/hirsutism
Breasts/galactorrhoea
Acne
Gynaecological examination

    —vulva, vagina, cervix, uterus, adnexae

A rapid scheme for the diagnosis of amenorrhea is shown as a flow chart in Fig. 7.1. Minimal laboratory examinations are required in this scheme as endogenous oestrogen production can be estimated by a progestin withdrawal test in the case of amenorrhoea. This is unnecessary if oligo- rather than amenorrhoea is the presenting complaint. This leaves only prolactin to be measured and, in the case of a negative progestin withdrawal, FSH concentrations are measured to find out if the problem is hypogonadotrophic or hypergonadotrophic hypogonadism. An outflow tract defect can be diagnosed if both progestin and oestrogen/progestin withdrawal do not produce bleeding and FSH levels are in the normal range.

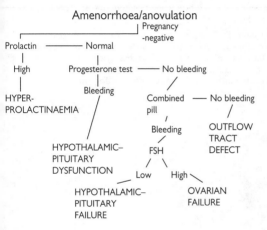

Fig. 7.1 A rapid scheme for the diagnosis of amenorrhoea/anovulation.

Once the type of amenorrhea has been classified in this way, a 2° round of investigation may be initiated, e.g.

- Hypothalamic–pituitary failure—test for anosmia, systemic diseases, 2° sex characteristics, weight loss.
- Hypothalamic–pituitary dysfunction—this group is further examined as for oligomenorrhoeic patients (see Fig. 7.2).
- Ovarian failure—karyotype, autoimmune antibodies.
- Hyperprolactinaemia—TSH, MRI of pituitary region.
- Outflow tract defect—pelvic ultrasound examination, karyotype if uterus is absent.

If oligomenorrhea is the presenting symptom, the scheme illustrated in Fig. 7.2 will be helpful.

In any of these situations, the aim is to arrive at a correct diagnosis for the cause of the oligo/amenorrhoea in the minimum amount of time and with a minimum of investigations. As this classification is very much treatment orientated, once the diagnosis is made it will indicate what is the correct treatment suitable for that specific diagnosis.

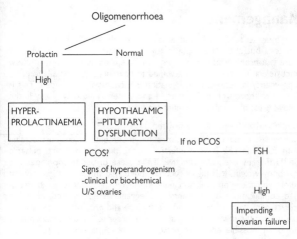

Fig. 7.2 Investigations of oligomenorrhoea.

Management

The treatment of oligo- and amenorrhoea depends not only on the aetiology but also on the purpose of the treatment, basically whether there is a problem of infertility or not. Except for women with outflow tract defect, the rest may be assumed to have oligo- or anovulation and, if pregnancy is desired, then ovulation induction will be needed. This is dealt with thoroughly in Chapter 14 and is mentioned only briefly in the following list of possible treatment modes.

Hypothalamic–pituitary failure

For ovulation induction, gonadotrophin treatment, which must contain both FSH and LH, is very effective. If the pituitary is intact, pulsatile GnRH therapy is equally effective. If the cause of the amenorrhoea is a low body weight, it is highly recommended that the patient gain weight before embarking on ovulation induction therapy in order to avoid associated complications of pregnancy. If pregnancy is not wanted, hormone replacement therapy (HRT) with oestrogens and progesterone, similar to that used in the menopause, is called for in order to avoid osteoporosis or any other possible effects of prolonged hypo-oestrogenism. Referral to tertiary care is recommended.

Hypothalamic–pituitary dysfunction

For women diagnosed as having PCOS and suffering infertility, the full range of possible treatments for ovulation induction is described in Chapter 5. These include weight loss, clomifene citrate, metformin and other insulin sensitizers, and low-dose gonadotrophin therapy.

For those who have PCOS but for whom infertility is not the presenting complaint, several options are open and may be tailored to the individual case.
- Weight loss is an essential first step for the overweight or frankly obese. A loss of just 5% or more of body weight may be enough to restore ovulation and menstruation.
- For those suffering from symptoms of hyperandrogenism (hirsutism, acne, alopecia), a combination of the anti-androgen cyproterone acetate (CPA) and ethinylestradiol (EE) is probably the most widely used treatment. CPA has an anti-androgen action at several sites: (1) in combination with EE, suppression of LH release by the anterior pituitary; (2) competition for the androgen receptor which it blocks; (3) as a progestogen in suppressing the action of 5α-reductase; and (4) with EE, increases SHBG concentrations. The combination of CPA (2mg/day) and EE (35 micrograms/day) (co-cyprindiol) given cyclically has proven very effective in the treatment of hirsutism and acne, as well as serving to restore regular menstruation and providing contraception. An impressive reduction in the degree of hirsutism occurs after 9 months of treatment, and acne has been successfully treated in almost 100% of cases using this minimal dose. The addition of CPA in a dose of 10–100mg/day on the first 10 days of the combined medication has proven effective for more severe cases. Patients need to be informed that this treatment is not 'instant', and that at least

4–9 months are needed to see an improvement in hirsutism and 3–5 months for acne, whereas menstruation is restored following the first treatment cycle. Further details and those of other anti-androgen preparations can be found in Chapter 6.

- Metformin, an oral insulin-lowering and anti-diabetic agent, has also been found to be reasonably effective in restoring ovulation and regular menstruation in women with PCOS. It is given in a dose of 1500–2500mg daily in divided daily doses. See Chapter 14 for further details.

Ovarian failure

For patients desiring pregnancy, ovum donation is the only successful option. Otherwise, HRT, as for menopausal patients, is recommended.

Hyperprolactinaemia

When hyperprolactinaemia and oligo- or amenorrhoea are associated with medication, the benefits and disadvantages of reducing the dosage or withdrawing medication must be carefully weighed up. Hypothyroidism as a cause should be treated with the appropriate medication for correction of thyroid function rather than with specific prolactin-lowering agents. All other cases of hyperprolactinaemia associated with ovulatory dysfunction and oligo/amenorrhoea, whether idiopathic or from a pituitary tumour, require treatment.

Neurosurgical treatment for hyperprolactinaemia is, today, very rarely required. For both micro- and macroprolactinomas, prolactin-lowering drugs are safer, more efficient and often capable of causing tumour shrinkage without recourse to surgery. Surgery should be reserved only for the very rare case completely resistant to medication, for non-secreting pituitary adenomas or para-sellar tumours, and in those who have severe visual disturbances which fail to improve with medication. For all the rest, prolactin-lowering medication will serve the purpose adequately.

Many dopamine agonists are in use for the treatment of infertility associated with hyperprolactinaemia.

- Bromocriptine is the most widely used dopamine agonist. Provided in tablets of 2.5mg, it is wise to start with half a tablet, at bedtime, taken with toast or a dry biscuit, for the first week to 10 days of treatment. This tends to help avoid the rather unpleasant, not infrequent side-effects of this drug, i.e. nausea, vomiting, diarrhoea and postural hypotension. Following this initial dosage regime, 2.5mg nightly can be given, which may be titrated up to a maximum dose of even 20mg/day, but this is rarely needed for restoration of ovulation and menstruation. The best way of gauging the dose is restoration of regular menstruation. This is a better indication than the serum prolactin concentration that the correct dose is being administered. Follow-up of tumour size by MRI or CT is only really needed when no response is seen either by the return of regular ovulation or at least by a reduction in serum prolactin concentrations. Restoration of menstruation is achieved in ~85% of cases, even including those with a macroprolactinoma. This is a remarkably successful and simple treatment and has the additional advantage that it is capable of reducing the size of the prolactinomata and, often, with continued treatment, microprolactinomata will disappear altogether.

- Cabergoline is at the least equally as effective as bromocriptine and has the added advantage that it is long acting. A single oral dose can lower prolactin concentrations for 1–2 weeks. For the resumption of ovulatory cycles, the recommended dose is 0.5–2mg/week, usually divided into a twice-weekly dosage.
- Quinagolide, in contrast to the above, is a non-ergot derivative and seems, for that reason, to have fewer side-effects than the ergot derivatives referred to above. The starting dose is 25 micrograms for the first 3 days followed by 50 micrograms for 3 days and then 75 micrograms daily.

Outflow tract defects

Imperforate hymen and transverse vaginal septa are treated with relatively simple surgical techniques to restore the integrity of the outflow tract. Imperforate hymen is probably the most frequent obstructive anomaly of the female genital tract, but estimates of its frequency vary from 1 case per 1000 population to 1 case per 10 000 population.

The diagnosis is sometimes made in infancy, with the infant noted to have a bulging, yellow-grey mass at or beyond the introitus. More commonly it presents at puberty with cyclical pelvic/abdominal pain and amenorrhoea. Treatment is via cruciate incision in the hymen.

Restoration of endometrial function, damaged by intra-uterine adhesions or overzealous curettage, is more complicated and less successful. Operative hysteroscopy to remove adhesions is the most popular option. Insertion of an intra-uterine contraceptive device for 3–6 months has also met with some success. Both these treatment modes are usually supported by a course of antibiotics and oestrogens.

Menopause and hormone replacement therapy

Introduction

The term menopause is derived from the Greek *menos* (month) and *pauses* (cessation), but the term has come to be used to describe the climacteric, which again is derived form the Greek *klimakter* (rung of ladder).

The average age at which the menopause occurs has not changed, but life expectancy has improved to the extent that in the UK women can expect to spend about one-third of their lives in a menopausal state.

- *Menopause*: defined retrospectively 1yr after last menstrual period; average age 51.
- *Climacteric*: the 'climb' to the menopause; average age 45–47 (lasting 4yrs on average—up to 10yrs).
- *Early menopause*: <45yrs.
- *Premature ovarian failure*: <40yrs.

Pathophysiology

The number of primordial follicles that a female has `shrinks throughout life, with their being no replacement.

- Newborn   2 milllion
- Puberty   300 000–400 000
- 40yrs+   Few thousand
- Postmenopause   Few or no ova

The number of ovarian follicles available to mature each cycle is depleted (300–400 cycles on average) as the women get older. As one oocyte ovulates, ~1000 become atretic through apoptosis. There are two critical landmarks in the ovarian failure process: the first is a marked decline in fertility (no cycle dysfunction) and the second occurs when the menstrual cycle changes become noticeable, with a shortened follicular phase and luteal dysfunction.

The effect of the reduced pool of follicle for stimulation is that the oestrogen levels start to fall. Initially there is a 'compensated failure'. This is then associated with an increase in the production of FSH and a decrease in the level of inhibin produced by the follicles. Early follicular inhibin B and FSH appear to be predictive of ovarian reserve/response to gonadotrophin stimulation. The FSH level will, however, vary in the climacteric with a non-linear increase, and currently we are awaiting more population data on inhibin B. Due to the lack of more population data on inhibin B, the standard test remains FSH alone. 'Decompensated failure' occurs when the follicle pool is very low. FSH rises further (10- to 20-fold); LH rises 3-fold (shorter half-life). Oestrogen levels drop due to reduction in follicle number and qualitative effect on granulosa cell ageing. There is a permanent cessation of progesterone production; this can lead to endometrial proliferation and hyperplasia.

In the developed world, there is an increasing female life expectancy but unaltered age of menopause.

Other hormonal changes

Adrenal and ovarian androgens (testosterone and androstendione) decline. Some testosterone is still, however, produced by theca cells. Ovarian androstenedione production drops by half in menopause so that the majority is from the adrenals (1:4 ratio).

Sex hormone-binding globulin (SHBG) decreases due to reduction in ovarian oestradiol. The main postmenopausal oestrogen is oestrone. It is produced mainly in peripheral adipose tissue and postmenopausal ovary by aromatization of adrenal androstenedione. The amount of oestrone produced is related to body weight and age. Glucocorticoid administration in postmenopausal women will suppresses oestrogen production, confirming that it is from an adrenal production site.

Insulin resistance rises after the menopause. This change results in an increase in central adiposity (android rather than gynaecoid shape) and a decreased lean body mass.

Symptoms

The characteristic symptoms of the menopause include:

Acute	Intermediate/late
Hot flushes (70%)	Dyspareunia
Night sweats (70%)	Loss of libido
Insomnia	Urethral syndrome
Anxiety/irritability	Vaginal atrophy
Memory loss	
Poor concentration	
Mood changes	

Hot flushes

The hot flush, although it may characteristically start over the face or neck area, involves the whole body and is often followed by intense sweating and then by shivering (see figure 8.1). Hot flushes occur in 70% of Caucasian and Afro-Caribbean women but is less common in Japanese and Chinese; this may be cultural or possibly due to a high isoflavone diet.

Hot flushes are not present in Turner's or lifelong hypothalamic amenorrhoea patients, and obese women are partially protected probably due to their high oestrone production and lower SHBG levels. It is thought that the mechanism is such that: oestrogen induces hypothalamic opioid activity; the loss of this activity can lead to thermo-dysregulation, mediated by noradrenaline. Oestrogen also increases $\alpha 2$ adrenergic activity, hence the rationale for clonidine therapy.

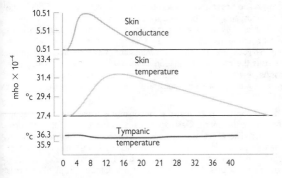

Fig. 8.1 Physiology of the hot flush. From Tataryn IV, Lomax P, Bajorek JG, Chesarek W, Meldrum DR, Judd HL. Postmenopausal hot flushes: a disorder of thermoregulation. *Maturitas* 1980; **2**: 101–107.

CNS systems

Oestrogen and progesterone receptors are co-located in the CNS in the hypothalamus, amygdala, preoptic area, hippocampus and the cerebellum. In these areas they mediate genomic effects, e.g. limbic system functions subserving emotion and behaviour. Oestrogen has a direct effect on 5-hydroxytryptamine (5-HT; serotonin) and noradrenaline receptors. It increases the rate of degradation of monoamine oxidase (MAO) thus increasing levels of 5-HT. Oestrogen also displaces tryptophan from albumin, providing more 5-HT substrate as well as enhancing the transport of 5-HT.

The depression that is seen at the menopause is partly due to serotonin and noradrenaline deficit. Oestrogen increases the levels of these neurotransmitters. The effect of oestrogen supplement in the form of HRT at the menopause on cognitive function is unclear. Some trials indicate that oestrogen improves function, as indicated by memory and attention improvements. Current evidence from randomized controlled trials (RCTs) is inadequate.

Urogenital

Women may experience a number of symptoms arising from the urogenital system around the menopause.

Vaginal symptoms	Urinary symptoms
Vaginal dryness, irritation, discharge	Recurrent urinary tract infections
Vulvo-vaginal pruritus, pain	Urinary frequency, urgency
Dyspareunia	Dysuria, voiding difficulties
Postcoital bleeding	Urinary incontinence
Prolapse	
Anorgasmia	

Most of these symptoms are a result of atrophy of vaginal and urethral epithelium (oestrogen receptors) with loss of rugations and stenosis. A decreased maturation of cells leads to a decreased number of superficial cells. There is a disturbance of the vaginal flora (decreased lactobacilli, increased faecal flora) and a resultant increase in vaginal pH. In the peri-urethral connective tissue there is a decreased amount of collagen.

Skeletal system

Bone mass reaches a peak in women towards the end of their third decade (see figure 8.2). It then remains relatively stable until the menopause, after which the loss is lifelong. 70% of women over the age of 80 will have measurable osteoporosis. It is estimated that there are some 60 000 hip fractures, 50 000 Colles fractures and 40 000 clinically apparent vertebral fractures a year in the UK.

Factors that can affect the bone mass include
- Affecting peak bone mass.
  - genetic/racial.
  - diet/calcium in adolescence.
- Affecting bone loss.
  - premature menopause.
  - amenorrhoea.
  - exercise/diet/weight.
  - smoking/alcohol/caffeine.
  - use of corticosteroids.

Risk factors that may affect the chance of fracture include

- Low bone mass.
  - low body weight.
  - current cigarette smoking.
- Personal or family history of fracture.
- Risk factors for falls.
  - confusion disorders.
  - medications (sedative hypnotics, alcohol).
  - neuromuscular disease.
  - environmental factors.

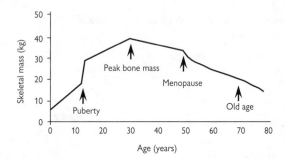

Fig. 8.2 Bone density in women. Adapted from Birdwood 1996.

Cardiovascular risk

Coronary heart disease (CHD) is uncommon among premenopausal women, particularly if they do not smoke. There is a rapid increase in the risk following the menopause, and cardiovascular disease is now a leading cause of death among postmenopausal women. The mechanism whereby premenopausal women have protection against CHD is not clear; however, it is known that oestrogen has a number of protective effects including:

• Nitric oxide-mediated vascular dilatation.
• Inhibition of platelet aggregation.
• Increased high-denstiy lipoprotein (HDL), decreased low-denstiy lipoprotein (LDL).
• Reduction in insulin resistance.
• Antioxidant effect on endothelial cells.
• Reduction in myocardial ischaemia.

The reduction in this increased risk of CHD in women on HRT after the menopause was addressed in two large studies discussed in detail below.

'Women's Health Initiative (WHI) trial' and 'Million Women Study'

The WHI trial was set up with the primary aim to test whether post-menopausal use of HRT protected women from CHD. The study was an RCT which enrolled >16 000 American women. The women were randomized to take HRT in the form of 0.625mg of conjugated equine oestrogens and 2.5mg of medroxyprogesterone acetate daily, or a placebo. After 5yrs of follow-up, the women on HRT were found to have:

- Higher incidence of breast cancer.
- Higher incidence of myocardial infarction, stroke and pulmonary embolus.
- Lower CHD risk in 50–59yr age group women.
- Decreased incidence of hip fractures and colorectal cancers.

Million Women Study. This was a UK-based study that collected data from women attending breast screening as part of the NHS breast screening programme. One million women were followed between May 1996 and March 2001. The women were aged between 50 and 64. Half of the women used HRT at some point, with half of those taking the combined hormone medication. Results of this study showed:

- Combined oestrogen/gestagen HRT was associated with a 2-fold increase in breast cancer when compared with non-users.
- Use of oestrogen-only HRT represented a 30% increased risk of breast cancer.
- Looking at a 10yr period, the risk of breast cancer is four times greater in those taking a combined HRT than an oestrogen-only preparation.

UK Committee on the Safety of Medicines and HRT

Following publication of these two significant studies, the UK Committee on the Safety of Medicines issued advice to prescribers of HRT. This advise can be summarized as follows:

- For short-term (e.g. 2–3yrs) use of HRT for the relief of menopausal symptoms, the benefits outweigh the risks for most women.
- Longer term use of HRT is licensed for the prevention of osteoporosis. However, patients should be aware of the increased incidence of some conditions with long-term HRT use and of alternative options for the prevention of osteoporosis.
- The decision to use HRT should be discussed with each woman on an individual basis, taking into account her history, risk factors and personal preferences .
- Individual risks and benefits should be regularly reappraised (e.g. at least annually) whilst using HRT.
- HRT should not be used for the prevention of CHD.

HRT preparations

Oestrogens are effective at relieving menopausal symptoms. For all women who have not had a hysterectomy, a progestogen should be added for at least 10 days of each month to prevent endometrial hyperplasia and carcinoma. The routes of administration of the oestogen can be:

- oral.
- patches.
- implants.
- vaginal rings.
- gel.
- nasal spray.

Oral regimens are well tolerated by many women, are cheaper and are an appropriate first choice. Oestrogen is given continuously, with progestogen added for at least 10 days per cycle, in women with an intact uterus. Fixed-dose combination preparations are convenient for patients not experiencing adverse effects and may improve compliance. Adjustment of dose of individual hormones is possible by prescribing oestrogen and progestogen separately, or by using combination packs with varying strengths. Oral regimens do, however, deliver a high level of oestrogen to the liver with an increased risk of gallstone formation and a tendency to increase triglyceride formation.

Transdermal regimens women who experience nausea on oral therapy may tolerate a 'patch' better. Transdermal regimens may also be considered for women with raised plasma triglycerides, gallbladder disease or poor absorption. They are more expensive than oral regimens. Topical preparations containing oestrogen alone or containing estradiol in combination with norethisterone or medroxyprogesterone are available

Estradiol subcutaneous implants provide a depot oestrogen effect that lasts 4–12 months. Oral progestogen will also be required if the woman has an intact uterus. Estradiol levels should be monitored before a new implant is inserted.

Vaginal preparations: vaginal oestrogen creams and pessaries are indicated for short-term use for atrophic vaginitis. They do not prevent osteoporosis. Long-term use by the vaginal route may be associated with endometrial hyperplasia, and additional oral progestogen should be given, perhaps quarterly.

Regimens

The sequential regimens have oestrogen in the first half of a 28-day cycle with progestogen in the second half. This is the appropriate regimen for women in the perimenopausal state. Continuous combined therapy which has progestogen every day is useful for those women who are a few years past the menopause and do not wish to have any vaginal bleeding.

Table 8.1 Suggested regimens

Perimenopausal women:	Oral or transdermal cyclic oestrogen plus cyclic progestogen
Non-smoking perimenopausal women requiring contraception:	Low dose oral contraceptive until menopause, then HRT
Women 2–3yrs postmenopause:	Continuous oestrogen–progestogen—oral or transdermal
Women remaining symptomatic on adequate doses of oral HRT:	Transdermal oestrogen plus progestogen
Women who have had a hysterectomy:	Continuous oestrogen alone—oral or transdermal

Side-effects and complications of HRT

The main side-effect is vaginal bleeding in women with a uterus. This can be decreased by the use of a continuous combined therapy in women 2–3yrs after the menopause. The addition of progestogen in women with a uterus can cause bloating, fluid retention and mastalgia. Progestogens can be administered vaginally as a gel or pessary to try and reduce the severity of any side-effects.

Venous thrombosis: There is a very small increased risk of venous thrombosis in women on HRT who do not have a previous history of venous thrombosis. The absolute risk has been approximated to 2/10 000 treatment years for venous thrombosis, 0.6/10 000 treatment years for pulmonary embolus and 2/million treatment years for death. The first 12 months of treatment are associated with the highest risk.

Breast disease: The evidence for an increase in breast cancer is indicated above (WHI and Million Women Study). HRT should be avoided in those with a family history of a first-degree relative with breast cancer. HRT also increases the incidence of benign mastalgia and mammographic density. As a result of this, HRT can lead to an increase in psychological and surgical morbidity because of the increased number of mammographically guided or open breast biopsies that have to be performed.

Alternative treatment

- Norethisterone 5mg has been shown to be effective in reducing hot flushes and sweats, but it has little effect on other menopausal systems. Medroxyprogesterone acetate and megestrol may work similarly.
- Propranolol and clonidine have been used for the treatment of hot flushes, but the effect is probably no better than placebo.
- Vaginal oestrogen preparations can be used to treat atrophic vaginitis, but repeated use can lead to systematic absorption.
- Selective oestrogen receptor modulators (SERMS) are effective in the prevention of bone loss and reduce the incidence of breast cancer. They may increase hot flushes slightly.
- Naturally occurring oestrogens such as phytoestrogens occur in cereals and vegetables. Pharmaceutical preparations of these phytoestrogens have not been shown to be any better than placebo.

Further reading and information

Rees M, Purdie J. *Management of the Menopause: The Handbook*, 4th edn. London: Royal Society of Medicine Press Ltd, 2006.
The British Menopause Society: http://www.thebms.org.uk/index.php.

Initial advice to those concerned about delays in conception

Prevalence of fertility problems

Sixteen per cent of couples fail to conceive after 1yr of unprotected regular intercourse. After 2 years, with no treatment, about half of these will still not have conceived and, after a further year, ~7% in all will remain infertile. Most couples will turn for help after 1yr, depending on their particular culture. That means that one in seven couples will look for advice after 1yr.

.

Timing of the initial investigation

Couples who have not succeeded in conceiving after 1yr of regular unprotected intercourse should be offered investigation. Earlier investigation and treatment should be initiated where there is a history of obvious fertility-impeding factors such as oligo/amenorrhoea, previous pelvic surgical intervention, previous ectopic pregnancy, pelvic inflammatory disease (PID), undescended testis, sexual dysfunction, a history of cancer treatment or if the female partner is aged ≥35yr. At all consultations both partners should be present if possible.

Female partner's age

Advancing female age is probably the single most important factor influencing fertility potential. Physiologically, from the age of ~35yrs onwards, there is a steady downward trend in fertility capacity, and this is probably a reflection of the declining number of primordial follicles remaining, biological ageing and exposure to many deleterious influences on the ova remaining in the ovaries. In addition to the persistently decreasing number of available, potentially fertilizable oocytes, it is also assumed that the best quality ova are preferentially recruited in the earlier stages of the reproductive period. As a result, from the mid-thirties onwards, fertility potential decreases considerably and, after the age of 42, a spontaneous pregnancy becomes quite a rare event. Advancing female age affects not only natural conception but also the results of ovulation induction and assisted reproductive technologies. Public awareness of these facts is insufficient. Many women, in this modern day and age of career women, delayed wish for conception, aspiring single mothers and increasing divorce rates and second marriages, do not comprehend the profound effect of advancing female age on fertility potential. We have not yet succeeded in impressing the general public sufficiently with these facts. An awareness of the declining pregnancy rates with age at least allows an informed consideration of the timing of attempted conception when this is flexible. In order to inform couples fully of their prognosis regarding fertility potential, especially if the female partner is in the more advanced age group, data on the state of ovarian function are needed. This information should be utilized not only to forecast the chances on conception but, not infrequently, to decide whether treatment should be embarked upon at all. To answer these questions, information regarding both the number of available oocytes (ovarian reserve) and their quality is needed. Tests of ovarian reserve include day 3 FSH and estradiol, inhibin B, anti-Mullerian hormone, antral follicle count and dynamic tests such as clomifene challenge test. The results of the tests available require accurate interpretation of their value before any informed discussion can be undertaken.

Frequency and timing of intercourse

Many couples attempting to conceive are unaware that regular intercourse around the time of ovulation is a basic requirement. Trite as this may sound, a simple explanation regarding the approximate time of presumed ovulation for the woman with regular cycles may prove very helpful. If the couple are advised to have intercourse a minimum of once every 2 days around this time, pregnancies can be achieved in not a few cases without further investigation or treatment. It is true that this sort of advice may produce a stressful situation in some cases but, if so, this can be annulled. In general if couples are advised to have regular intercourse throughout the menstrual cycle (2–3 times per week) this may be more simply understood.

Environmental and dietary influences

- *Alcohol*—Excessive regular alcohol consumption by the male partner may affect not only sexual performance but also semen quality.
- *Smoking*—The habit of smoking is clearly not good for general health, and couples attempting to conceive should be encouraged to stop smoking. There is evidence to show that women who smoke heavily may have a reduced fertility potential and that the semen quality of men who smoke may be reduced.
- *Occupation*—The occupations of the couple concerned about their fertility should be noted. Occupations such as long-distance lorry or bus driving in hot climates, those involving exposure to bromide or similar chemicals, or work involving exposure to irradiation have all been associated with a decrease in fertility potential.
- *Medications*—Many medications, whether prescribed, over-the-counter or recreational drugs, may interfere with male and female infertility. Due note must be taken of such medication and appropriate measures taken. Some of the most common examples include some sedatives that increase prolactin discharge, so-called complementary medications containing oestrogens, and salazopyrines that may have drastic effects on semen quality.
- *Body weight*—Both extremes of body weight may have a significant effect on fertility potential. Obese women (BMI ≥30), especially those with associated anovulation, have a significant disadvantage in fertility potential, take longer to conceive, require more drugs for ovarian stimulation and are at a greater risk of miscarriage than those of normal weight. Participation in a programme involving instruction in diet, weight loss and exercise before the initiation of any further treatment can be very rewarding. Obese men are also more likely to have reduced fertility and should similarly be encouraged to lose weight. Underweight women (BMI <19) who have oligo- or amenorrhoea should be encouraged to increase their weight as, often, this alone may restore regular ovulation.
- *Folic acid supplementation*—Every woman intending to conceive should be advised to take folic acid, 400 micrograms/day, before conception and up to 12 weeks into the pregnancy. This has been shown significantly to reduce the risk of having a baby with a neural tube defect. For women who have previously had an infant with a neural tube defect or who are receiving anti-epileptic medication, a higher dose of 5mg/day is recommended.

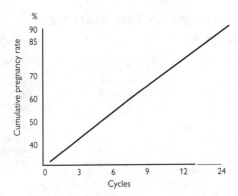

Fig. 10.1 Cumulative conception rates according to the number of cycles of attempted conception in the general population.

General points before starting investigation

- Infertility is the problem of a couple and, wherever possible, both members should be involved in clinic visits and decision making. Apportioning 'blame' to one or the other should be avoided.
- Infertility is a stressful situation. Sympathetic handling, full explanations and encouragement are an essential component of the management.
- A basic explanation of the timing of intercourse in relation to the probable time of ovulation can be very helpful to the couple.
- Overweight and obesity are obstacles in the attainment of a pregnancy and are also associated with an increased incidence of spontaneous miscarriage. Advice on the importance of these facts and the necessary information for their correction should be given before any treatment is initiated. Warnings about impairment of fertility function by excessive alcohol intake, cigarette smoking and drug abuse should also be given at this stage where relevant.
- Every woman attempting conception should be given folic acid, 0.4mg daily, in order to prevent neural tube defects in the infant. This should be continued until at least the 12th week of the pregnancy.
- Fertility potential in general starts to decline after the age of 35yrs in the female. Delay in the decision to conceive beyond this age, and especially over the age of 39, an increasing trend in the modern world, can create serious problems. Couples should be well informed of this situation when discussing decision making.

Investigation of fertility problems

Introduction

The aim of the investigation of the infertile couple is to find the cause(s) of the problem and treat accordingly. Both investigation and treatment are logical stepwise processes. A 'blunderbus' approach may sometimes be successful, but it is not the most efficient, safe and economical way to approach the problem.

Accurate history taking is absolutely essential for discerning the cause(s) of the infertility. By listening carefully and asking direct questions, many clues can be found. A suggested check-list for the female partner has been presented in Table 7.2. The headings can be used as a guide at the first consultation. The answers to the direct questions can prompt further more detailed inquiries, e.g. is the amenorrhoea 1° or 2°? If 1°, is there a problem with the sense of smell. If 2°, are there any hot flushes, etc.?.

A thorough gynaecological and general examination should also be performed at the first visit. Again, a suggested check-list is provided in Table 7.1. For history taking and examination of the male partner, see below.

The results of the history and examination alone will often indicate the possible cause of the infertility and will also dictate the order in which the more specific examinations be made. It should be remembered that many couples may have more than one specific cause for their infertility and also that up to 30% may be 'unexplained' in that all the basic, and more specific, infertility investigations prove to be normal.

The investigation of the infertile couple at a basic, first-line level involves a semen analysis, and an examination of ovulatory function and of the integrity of the female reproductive tract. An abnormal result for any of these basic investigations may prompt second-line examinations. Table 11.1 sets out possible first- and second-line examinations which are used commonly.

Table 11.1 Possible first- and second-line examinations for the investigation of fertility

	Ovulation	Mechanical	Male
First-line	Mid-luteal progesterone (BBT, U/S, urinary LH)	HSG	Semen analysis
Second-line	Day 3 FSH, LH, T, PROL Androgens, in serum	Laparoscopy Hysteroscopy Tubal catheter	Physical Exam. Hormones Venous flow

Investigation of the male partner

A semen analysis should be performed in every case of infertility as a routine screening test. The semen is produced by masturbation and the fresh sperm should be examined within 30min. It has become traditional to request abstinence from ejaculation for 2–3 days before obtaining the sample. Abstinence of >5 days before sampling may result in decreased sperm motility.

Normal parameters of a semen sample are listed in Table 11.2. The standard criteria are those of the WHO (2000), but for the analysis of sperm morphology Kruger's strict criteria are now widely used and have been added. Sperm motility is graded according to progressive forward motility, grade a (≥25% rapid progressive motility) or grade b (slow or sluggish progressive motility) or, alternatively, from grade I, fast forward, grade II, slow forward, grade III, minimal forward progression, to grade IV, no motility.

A reduced sperm concentration, oligospermia, is often accompanied by reduced sperm motility, asthenospermia. More detailed information regarding sperm motility can be obtained by using a computerized image analysis system which is said to correlate well with the fertilizing capacity of the sperm. Kruger's strict criteria are recommended for the assessment of sperm morphology. According to these criteria, <4% normal forms, teratozoospermia, carries a poor prognosis for fertilization.

A completely normal semen analysis does not require a further examination and, practically, does not require any further investigation of the male partner. An abnormal semen analysis demands a repeat examination, best done 3 months later, before any therapeutic decisions are made as a single-sample analysis will falsely identify ~10% of men as abnormal, but repeating the test reduces this to 2%.

Theoretically, a full history and examination of the male partner should be taken at the first clinic visit. In practice, obviously relevant history (e.g. undescended testis, orchitis) is noted at this time, but the rest of the detailed history and physical examination is usually only performed following an abnormal semen analysis.

Table 11.2 WHO reference values for semen analysis, 2000: normal parameters of a semen sample

Volume: 2.0mL or more
Liquefaction time: Within 60 minutes
pH: 7.2 or more
Concentration: 20 million spermatozoa/mL or more
Total sperm number: 40 million spermatozoa per ejaculate or more
Motility: 50% or more (grades a* and b**) or 25% with progressive forward motility (grade a*)
Vitality: 75% or more live
White blood cells: fewer than 1 million/mL
Morphology: >30% normal forms (WHO)   >14% normal forms (Kruger strict criteria)

* Grade a = rapid progressive motility (sperm moving swiftly, usually in a straight line).
** Grade b b= slow or sluggish progressive motility (sperm may be less linear in their progression).

History

- Medical—onset of puberty, diabetes mellitus, cystic fibrosis, past history of mumps, orchitis, STDs. Anosmia.
- Surgical—maldescended testis, hernia repair, varicocoele.
- Family history—genetic diseases.
- Medications—including anabolic steroids.
- Occupation—exposure to excessive heat, chemicals, excessive physical activity.
- Abuse—drugs, alcohol, smoking.

Examination

- Androgenicity—hair distribution, voice, body build, gynaecomastia.
- Testicular size—if abnormal can be quantified with an orchidometer (Prader beads). The normal range is 12–30mL. Testicular consistency.
- Undescended testis, spermatocoele, varicocoele, absence of the vas deferens.
- Rectal examination—palpation of the prostate gland, prostatic massage to obtain a urethral secretion for culture.

Further examinations

- Hormonal—serum concentrations of LH, FSH, testosterone, estradiol and prolactin. Hormone concentrations are principally of use for confirming suspected diagnoses of hypogonadotrophic hypogonadism (very low gonadotrophins) or of testicular failure when gonadotrophins are high and testosterone low.
- Chromosome analysis—Klinefelter's syndrome (47, XXY) should be suspected if the testes are small and firm.

- Imaging of the testes—ultrasound, isotopic examination of testicular blood flow for a suspected varicocoele, vasogram if there is a suspicion of obstructive azospermia (normal sized testes with normal hormonal concentrations).
- Postcoital test (PCT)—a PCT, performed during the immediate preovulatory period ~10h after intercourse, entails examining retrieved cervical mucous under a microscope for the presence and movement of sperm. It is only really useful when positive, i.e. the presence of ≥10 motile sperm per microscopic low-power field is reassuring that intercourse is successfully depositing motile sperm in receptive cervical mucous. A complete absence of sperm could indicate a faulty coital technique, azospermia or hostile cervical mucous. The absence of sperm motility could indicate a hostile cervical mucous or asthenospermia. Many units no longer employ the PCT as a routine examination due to its limited yield of useful information.

The management of male factor infertility can be found in Chapter 13 with information on intra-uterine insemination in Chapter 17, intracytoplasmic sperm injection in Chapter 20 and donor insemination in Chapter 21.

Investigation of the female partner

The investigation of the female partner basically consists of an examination of ovulatory function and the mechanical integrity of the reproductive tract. While ovulatory function is relatively easy to assess, the investigation of a mechanical factor is more invasive and may be delayed unless there is a specific indication, e.g. a history of pelvic surgery, ectopic pregnancy, pelvic inflammatory disease (PID), endometriosis or appendicectomy.

Ovulatory function

Any form of menstrual irregularity, not within the limits of a 24–35 day cycle, strongly suggests a diagnosis of anovulation or oligo-ovulation. The converse is not always true as the occasional woman with regular cycles may be anovulatory. Painful menstruation usually indicates that ovulation is occurring. For confirmation that ovulation is occurring, four possible methods are in common use: plasma progesterone concentrations, a basal body temperature (BBT) chart, vaginal ultrasound examination and urinary LH kits.

- Plasma progesterone concentrations are arguably the most accurate way to estimate whether ovulation has occurred. For women with a regular cycle of 28 days, a plasma progesterone estimation on cycle day 20 or 21 of ≥8ng/mL (25nmol/L) will rule out a diagnosis of anovulation. If the usual cycle is 35 days in length, then this examination should be done around cycle day 28, i.e. ~7 days before the expected menstruation. For women with mild oligomenorrhoea (cycle length >35 days), progesterone can be measured on day 28 and then once a week until menstruation occurs. If periods only occur less than once every 2 months or in cases of 2° amenorrhoea, there is little point in hunting for progesterone estimations as the diagnosis of severe oligo- or anovulation is self-apparent.

- The principle of the BBT chart to estimate whether ovulation is occurring is that the secretion of progesterone following ovulation, into the circulation, will cause a rise in body temperature of ~0.5°C. The typical BBT chart will thus be biphasic, i.e. the temperature following ovulation will be higher than in the first part or follicular phase. The day before the temperature rise is usually denoted as the day of ovulation. Although the BBT is a simple, cheap and non-invasive screening test, it suffers from many inaccuracies, particularly false negatives, and is open to too much misinterpretation. It is very doubtful whether the BBT still has a place in the routine screening for ovulatory problems. Further, it has been found to be a niggling nuisance for many women as temperature must be measured every morning, immediately on waking.

- A vaginal ultrasound examination before and after ovulation should record a large developing dominant follicle which disappears following ovulation. In addition, most competent ultrasonographers are able to diagnose the presence of a corpus luteum if ovulation has occurred. This will be accompanied by a small amount of fluid in the pouch of Douglas.

Physical examination can give many clues as to the cause of anovulation. Most obvious at first glance is the weight of the patient. Weight and height should always be recorded, and the BMI calculated. This is done with the following formula:

$$BMI = \frac{Weight\ (kg)}{Height\ in\ metres^2}$$

A normal BMI is 20–25
<20 is underweight
25.1–30 is overweight
>30 is frank obesity.

Some geographical variations in these diagnoses exist. For example, in most South-East Asian communities, any BMI >25 is regarded as obesity.

Overweight and obesity
Overweight and obesity are often associated with PCOS, and in turn PCOS is often characterized by hirsutism and/or acne, both of which are easily discernible on examination. In cases of suspected PCOS who are obese, acanthosis nigricans, dark discoloration of the skin in the axillary or nuchal regions, is a tell-tale sign of insulin resistance. Waist circumference should be measured at the level between the umbilicus and the iliac crests in all overweight women as this again may be a good reflection of insulin resistance when >88cm.

Weight-related amenorrhoea
Women whose BMI is <20 may have irregular or absent ovulation due to so-called, weight-related amenorrhoea. This may be due to loss of weight due to dieting and to anorexia nervosa in its extreme. Direct questioning regarding diet, alcohol or drug abuse is mandatory.

Oestrogen deficiency
Physical examination can also reveal signs of oestrogen deficiency such as poor breast development, lack of development of the vulva, vaginal dryness and lack of additional 2° sexual characteristics. These signs indicating oestrogen deprivation could be due to either hypo- or hypergonadotrophic hypogonadism, when either is associated with 1° amenorrhoea. Although Turner's syndrome is rare as a cause of amenorrhoea, it can often be easily diagnosed by the typical body habitus; short stature, webbed neck, cubitus valgus and often a systolic cardiac murmur.

Distribution of hair growth
Distribution of hair growth should be noted. A male distribution would indicate hyperandrogenism and a lack of body hair could be a sign of androgen insensitivity. Clitoral enlargement or lack of development would be in parallel to these respective conditions in their extreme.

Once the diagnosis of oligo- or anovulation has been established, further investigation is required to find the cause. Full details of the classification of ovulatory disorders and their investigation are described in Chapter 7.

Investigation of a possible mechanical factor

X-ray hysterosalpingography (HSG)

If there is a previous history in the female partner of an STD, a complicated delivery, Caesarean section, previous ectopic pregnancy, PID, endometriosis or surgical interventions in the pelvic region, including appendicectomy, a screening test, usually X-ray HSG, should be performed. An HSG should also be performed if both semen analysis and ovulatory function are normal.

The HSG is a diagnostic procedure in which there is radiographic visualization of the cervical canal, uterine cavity and lumina of the fallopian tubes by the injection of radio-opaque contrast medium through a cervical cannula. It is capable of demonstrating congenital uterine abnormalities, intra-uterine lesions such as polyps, fibroids and adhesions, and patency and abnormalities of the fallopian tubes.

Iodine sensitivity is a contraindication. An HSG should not be performed during uterine bleeding, to avoid intravasation, and not in the luteal phase of the cycle, to avoid the possible presence of an early pregnancy. Water-soluble media are now used in preference to oil-based media as the latter carry a risk of intravasation and possible embolism. The injection of up to 5mL of contrast medium, usually water-soluble, is often enough to obtain all the information needed. The use of larger than necessary volumes may produce discomfort and may also obscure lesions in the uterine cavity.

The demonstration of a normal uterine cavity on HSG obviates the need for hysteroscopy, which may be employed for the confirmation and possible operative removal of lesions within the uterine cavity demonstrated on HSG. Some centres use laparoscopy as a screening test if the history is suggestive of a possible mechanical factor, but HSG serves this purpose well and is certainly a less invasive technique. If HSG is suggestive of a tubal lesion or peritubal adhesions, or when significant pelvic adhesions are suspected, then a laparoscopy is performed.

If the HSG confirms tubal patency and a normal uterine cavity, then no further work-up to diagnose a mechanical factor cause of the infertility is usually needed at the screening stage. Abnormal findings in the HSG will dictate what further steps are to be taken. These may include a diagnostic laparoscopy and hysteroscopy which may be diagnostic or operative, or gross tubal damage demonstrated on the HSG, such as sactosalpinx, may indicate direct progress to IVF.

Although HSG should be used as a purely diagnostic procedure, there is some evidence of a possible therapeutic effect in patients with apparently normal patent fallopian tubes. Following an HSG with water-soluble contrast medium, more pregnancies result than would be expected to occur spontaneously when not performing an HSG. This may be due to the separation of 'sticky' fimbria, mild peritubal adhesions or tubal plugs. In addition, selective salpingography and treatment of proximal tubal occlusive disease can be performed at the same time as the original diagnostic test.

Ultrasound

Sonohysterography is the infusion of saline into the uterus during sono-graphy. It is simple, cheap, minimally invasive, relatively painless and avoids the use of hysteroscopy or radiation for obtaining information principally about the uterine cavity. However, due to the limitations of sonohystero-graphy, mainly its inability to visualize tubal patency directly, HSG remains the gold standard for routine screening for infertility and hysteroscopy for direct visualization of the uterine cavity. Sonosalpingography, employing a contrast medium, despite initial enthusiasm, has fallen from grace for various reasons.

Laparoscopy

Laparoscopy entails the controlled introduction of carbon dioxide into the peritoneal cavity in order to distend it and enable visualization by the introduction of the fibre-optic laparoscope. For the investigation of infer-tility, a blue dye is injected through the cervical canal in order to assess tubal patency and free flow into the pelvic cavity.

A full assessment of the pelvis should be made on laparoscopy, including the peritoneal surface of the uterus, bladder, appendix and bowel. Endome-triosis can be spotted and mapped, and an inspection of the ovaries can reveal the presence of cysts, polycystic ovaries, normally developing follicles and signs of ovulation. Following a thorough inspection of the pelvis, blue dye is injected through a cervical cannula and evidence of its passage from both distal ends of the tubes should be sought as well as its free flow into the pelvic cavity. The presence of pelvic adhesions can be noted and, if thin and flimsy, they can easily be separated during the diagnostic procedure.

The advantages of laparoscopy and dye injection over HSG as a diagnostic procedure are that laparoscopy allows full visualization of the pelvic cavity and can diagnose the presence of endometriosis, pelvic adhesions, particu-larly peritubal and para-ovarian adhesions, and other pelvic pathology. Furthermore, some of these conditions can be treated during the same procedure. Laparoscopy is also usually capable of overcoming tubal spasm which is sometimes a cause of a false diagnosis of proximal tubal occlusion on HSG. However, laparoscopy cannot give information on the uterine cavity and, for this reason, many units combine a diagnostic laparoscopy with hysteroscopy at the same sitting.

The disadvantages of laparoscopy are that it is an invasive procedure which may cause morbidity such as anaesthetic complications, perforation of an abdominal viscus or haemorrhage. It also carries a 1:12 000 risk of mortality.

Although some centres employ laparoscopy as a first-line procedure for the investigation of infertility for patients thought to have co-morbidities, it is more commonly used for confirmation of abnormalities seen on HSG for clarifying so far unexplained infertility or for the diagnosis and extent of suspected endometriosis.

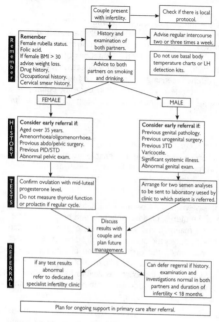

Fig. 11.1 Initial investigation of the couple at the primary care level.

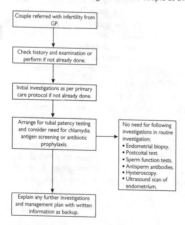

Fig. 11.2 Initial investigation and management of the couple in secondary care.

Further reading

Rowe PI, Comhaire FH, Hargreave TB, Mahmoud AM. *WHO Manual for the Standardized Investigation, Diagnosis and Management of the Infertile Male*. Cambridge: Cambridge University Press, 2000.

Collins JA. Diagnostic assessment of the infertile female partner. *Curr Probl Obstet Gynecol Fertil* 1988; **11**: 6–42.

Royal College of Obstetrician and Gynaecologists: fertility: assessment and treatment for people with fertility problems. February 2004 www.rcog.org.uk

Chapter 12

151

Management strategies for fertility problems

Principles

- People who have not conceived following 1yr of regular unprotected intercourse should be offered investigations.
- Earlier investigation may be offered when predisposing factors causing infertility become obvious from history-taking, e.g. oligo- or amenorrhoea, pelvic inflammatory disease (PID), pelvic surgery, endometriosis, ectopic pregnancy, undescended testis, etc., or when female age is ≥35yrs.
- Whenever possible, couples experiencing problems conceiving should be seen together, emphasizing the fact that the problem is that of a couple rather than an individual.
- Full explanations of investigations and treatment, with available additional counselling, can do much to alleviate the stress associated with fertility problems.
- The secondary management of infertility problems is a specialist subject and should ideally be performed in a dedicated centre with all the appropriate facilities.

Management of investigations

- The basic investigation of fertility problems should always include a semen analysis and assessment of ovulation.
- A normal semen analysis (see Table 11.2) precludes the need for further examination. A grossly abnormal result (azoospermia or severe oligo-terato-asthenospermia) demands a repeat test without further delay. An otherwise abnormal result should be confirmed or negated by a repeat test after 3 months as this is the normal duration of a sperm cycle. The practical help from the performance of a screening test for anti-sperm antibodies is doubtful. The further investigation of an abnormal semen analysis is described in detail in Chapter 11.
- Ovulation can be most simply confirmed in women with regular cycles by measuring serum progesterone concentration in the mid-luteal phase, i.e. day 21 in a woman with 28 day cycles. A serum progesterone concentration of >5ng/mL (25nmol/L) is a clear indication that ovulation is occurring. For women with prolonged cycles, a similar blood test should be performed ~7 days before the time of the expected menstruation. For women age ≥35yrs, a routine examination of serum FSH, estradiol and LH is warranted on day 3 of the cycle. For the further investigation of oligo- or anovulation, see Chapter 7.
- A history of conditions such as PID, pelvic surgery (including appendicectomy), previous Caesarean section, ectopic pregnancy, endometriosis, etc. indicates early investigation of a possible mechanical factor. In the absence of any hint of a mechanical problem, its assessment can be left to a later stage if needed, preferably by hysterosalpingography (HSG). Some prefer performing a laparoscopy using a dye as the first-line investigation, but this more invasive examination is often reserved for when an HSG reveals obvious abnormalities. Further, the use of an HSG as a screening test, as opposed to laparoscopy, has the advantage of demonstrating the uterine cavity and the fact that the revelation of clear evidence of a lesion, e.g. bilateral tubal occlusion with hydrosalpinges, can indicate proceeding directly to IVF or tubal surgery without the need to perform a diagnostic laparoscopy. For a more detailed discussion of investigation of a mechanical factor, see Chapter 11.

Management strategies

The basic history, examination and investigations will point to one or more diagnostic categories which will indicate the line of treatment to be employed. These are described only briefly here but more fully in the relevant individual chapters. Alternatively, no firm diagnosis may have been made following first- and second-line investigation (unexplained or idiopathic infertility) and this 'diagnosis', or lack of diagnosis, will be dealt with more fully below. Although divided here into male infertility, ovulatory and mechanical defects, it is not uncommon to unveil any combination of these, so-called multifactorial infertility. Similarly, the same line of treatment may be applied for different conditions.

Tables 12.1–12.4 list treatment possibilities according to the presumed diagnostic category and point out the relevant chapters containing detailed descriptions of the various treatment modes.

Male infertility

Table 12.1 lists possible treatment modes according to the various causes of sperm defects. This list is only a rough guide as, for example, the source of oligo-terato-asthenospermia is largely idiopathic and, in the majority of cases of male infertility, the sperm is treated rather than the man! Moreover, many of the treatment modes are suitable for different conditions and often the appropriate treatment is determined by the severity of the sperm defect rather than the underlying cause, whether known or not.

- The vast majority of sperm defects causing infertility are treated by either intra-uterine insemination (IUI) for the milder cases of oligo-terato-asthenospermia or intracytoplasmatic sperm injection (ICSI) for the rest.
- General health recommendations can, at best, only marginally improve sperm function, and the value of treatment with antibiotics for leucospermia and ligation of the spermatic vein(s) to repair varicocoele is still being disputed.
- The diagnoses of hypogonadotrophic hypogonadism and obstructive azoospermia are relatively rare, and together account for <3% of all cases of male infertility. In contrast, non-obstructive azoospermia and severe oligospermia due to testicular failure are common, and the cause is often unknown.

For details of the treatment modes listed in Table 12.1, the reader is referred to the relevant chapters indicated in the table.

- The high prevalence of unexplained infertility is a reminder of the lack of accuracy and subtlety of the diagnostic examinations employed. For example, tubal patency does not necessarily indicate normal tubal function, a normal routine semen examination tells us little about the functional capacity of the sperm and the subtleties of zona penetration, and proof of ovulation tells us nothing about the quality of the ovum.
- The decision of when to intervene for the treatment of unexplained infertility is influenced by the age of the female partner, the duration of infertility and the attitude adopted by both the physician and patients. After 1yr of unexplained infertility in a woman of ≥35yrs, no further delay in treatment intervention should be countenanced
- For women under the age of 35, particularly if they have children, expectant treatment for a further year (i.e. 2yrs infertility in all) seems reasonable. The decision of when to intervene is largely dictated by the mentality of the patients and the feeling that 'something' should be done.
- Table 12.4 lists possible treatment modes for unexplained infertility, all of which are necessarily empirical. They are listed in the usual order of going from the 'easy' to the more difficult. In practice, IUI alone or clomifene citrate alone fare only marginally better than expectant treatment. The combination of gonadotrophin stimulation and IUI is considerably more successful in terms of pregnancy rates. However, caution is advised regarding the high incidence of multiple pregnancies with this method. A full discussion can be found in Chapter 17.
- IVF is usually the last resort for these patients, usually after 3–6 cycles of stimulated cycles and IUI. IVF may uncover an explanation for the infertility by revealing a lack of fertilization due to either an egg or sperm defect, previously unsuspected.

Table 12.4 Treatment possibilities for unexplained infertility. (See also Chapters 17 and 18)

Expectant treatment
Clomifene citrate ± IUI
IUI—unstimulated cycle
IUI with gonadotrophin stimulation
IVF/ET

Male infertility

Introduction

Other than in cases of absolute azoospermia or severe oligosper-mia/asthenospermia, the impact of male factor on a couple's infertility is difficulty to quantify. Indeed, as can be seem in men after a vasectomy when extremely small amounts of motile sperm can be present, concep-tion can occur. Accepting this 'male factor' may be a contributing if not absolute factor in ~25% of cases of subfertility.

Aetiology

Primary testicular disease

The majority of cases of male factor lie in this category. In >50% of cases no obvious predisposing factor can be identified. Y chromosome micro-deletions are common in ~10–15% of men with azoospermia or severe oligospermia. These microdeletions are too small to be detected by karyotyping. They can be easily identified using polymerase chain reaction (PCR). Most of the microdeletions that cause azoospermia or oligospermia occur in the non-overlapping regions of the long arm of the Y chromsome. These regions, also called azoospermia factor regions, are responsible for spermatogenesis. The loci are termed AZFa, AZFb and AZFc from proximal to distal Yq (Yq11.21–23 region). Several genes located in AZF regions which are found to be associated with spermatogenesis are viewed as 'AZF candidate genes' (see figure 13.1).

Other causes of failure of spermatogenesis

- Testicular maldescent.
- Testicular torsion.
- Trauma or infection.
- Neoplasm of effect of chemotherapy.
- Haemosiderosis and Klinefelter's syndrome.
- Mumps and severe epididymo-orchitis are the main inflammatory causes.

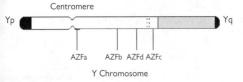

Fig. 13.1 The Y chromosome.

Obstructive male infertility

Obstruction can occur at any level of the male reproductive tract from the rete testis and the epididymis to the vas deferens. Obstruction can be due to congenital, inflammatory or iatrogenic causes. Congenital absence of the vas deferens is associated with carriers of cystic fibrosis (10% of cases) and thus pre-IVF screening for carrier status should be carried out.

Varicocoele

A varicocoele is the presence of abnormally tortuous viens of the pampiniform plexus within the spermatic cord. It is more common on the left that on the right, due to the direct insertion of the spermatic vein into the left renal vein. It occurs in both fertile and infertile males, but there appears to be a higher incidence in males with abnormal sperm parameters. The impact of a varicocoele on male fertility is controversial. It is argued by some that the varicocoele causes an increase in local temperature in the testis that inhibits spermatogenesis. However, radio-logical and surgical correction is thought not to improve sperm function, so this line of management is not commonly used.

Autoimmune causes

Approximately 12% of men have antisperm antibodies. This is significantly higher in men who have had trauma or surgery to the testis. Their presence may lead to a decrease in sperm motility and may impede sperm binding to the zona pellucida, although low levels are not thought to have any significant effect.

Endocrine causes

This is a rare cause, but will include hypogonadotrophic hypogonadism, thyroid and adrenal disease. Hyperprolactinaemia in men may lead to impotence but has little effect on sperm production.

Environmental factors

Exposure to heat, chemicals and ionizing irradiation can damage sperm production. The effects of environmental toxins on male infertility is unclear, although epidemiological studies have shown a decline in sperm quality in the developed or industrial world.

Drugs

Both medicinal and recreational drugs can affect sperm function, as shown in Table 13.1.

Table 13.1

Drug	Effect on spermatogenesis	Effect on sperm function
Anabolic steroid	Yes	No
Antifungal	Yes	No
Sulfasalazine	Yes	No
Corticosteroids	Yes	No
Alcohol	Yes	Yes
Cigarettes	Yes	Yes
Marijuana	Yes	Yes
Opiates	Yes	Yes
Chemotherapy drug	Permanent sterility	

Investigation of the male

Semen analysis

The large biological variability seen in the quality of sperm in repeated tests on the same individual limits the reproducibility of semen analysis as a diagnostic test. Table 13.2 shows the accepted value for a semen analysis.

Table 13.2 Normal and abnormal semen parameters

Semen characteristics	Normal	Borderline	Pathological
Volume (mL)	2.0–6.0	1.5–2.0	<1.5
Sperm concentration (million/mL)	20–250	10–20	<10
Total sperm count (million/ ejaculate)	>80	20–80	<20
Motility (0.5–2h after ejaculate)	>50	35–49	<35
Progression at 37°C (0–4)	3 or 4	2	<2
Vitality (% live)	≥75	50–74	<50
Morphology (/100 sperm)			
Head defects	<35	35–59	>60
Midpiece defects	≤20	21–25	>25
Tail defects	≤20	21–25	>25

Many other tests of semen quality have been devised. These include biochemical analysis of the seminal fluid and detection of antisperm antibodies. Biochemical analysis of the seminal fluid can provide information about the prostate, seminal vesicles and epididymis. The detection of antisperm antibodies using immunobeads or the mixed antibody reaction (MAR) test is still in the WHO criteria, with an MAR test of <50% sperm with adherent particles described as normal.

Sperm function tests

Routine semen analysis gives an indication of sperm function simply by the measure of normality or not. Some tests (Table 13.3) have been derived in order to try and measure sperm function as would occur *in vivo*. They are of academic interest as opposed to clinical.

Table 13.3 Sperm function tests

Hypo-osmotic swelling test
Test for sperm nuclear maturity
Measure of acrosome status
Acrosome reaction and acrosin activity
Hamster zona-free oocyte penetration
Human sperm–zona binding and penetration

Hormonal analysis of the male

The objective of hormonal analysis is to determine whether the azoo-spermia is due to primary testicular failure or an outflow obstruction. The normal gonadal–pituitary axis is shown in Fig. 13.2 and a flow diagram for investigation and diagnosis is shown in Fig. 13.3.

Hypogonadotrophic hypogonadism, often associated with Kallmann's syndrome, has been successfully treated with pulsatile GnRH or hMG to restore spermatogenic drive and hence fertility. Initiation of spermato-genesis can take several months.

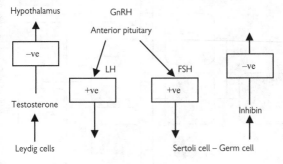

Fig. 13.2 The normal gonadal–pituitary axis.

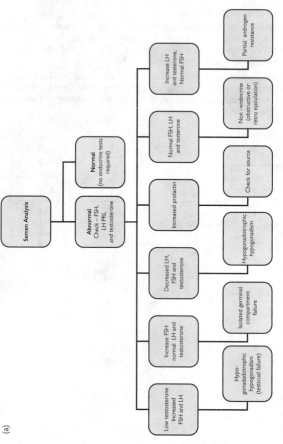

Fig. 13.3 Hormonal investigations (a) of males and (b) of hypogonadotrophic hypogonadism.

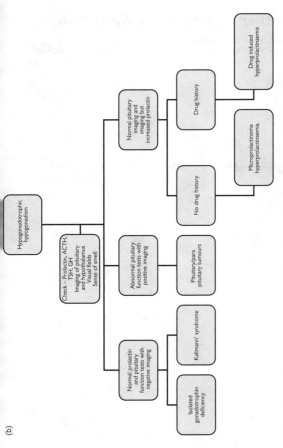

Fig. 13.3 (contd.) Hormonal investigations (a) of males and (b) of hypogonadotrophic hypogonadism.

(b)

Further reading and information

Infertility network UK: http://www.infertilitynetworkuk.com/index.php
European Society for Human Reproduction and Embryology: http://www.eshre.com/emc.asp

Ovulation induction

Introduction

Once the diagnosis of anovulation has been made and its cause determined (see Chapter 7), the starting treatment in that particular condition can also be determined.

The objective of ovulation induction is to restore the ovulatory state and reinstate fertility potential. This should, ideally, produce one ovulatory follicle and should not be confused with controlled ovarian stimulation for IVF or for IUI which is applied to already ovulating women with the aim of producing multiple ovulations.

The complications of ovulation induction are multiple pregnancies and ovarian hyperstimulation syndrome (OHSS). They are both caused by the induction of multiple follicular growth, are iatrogenic and largely preventable. Both can be avoided by expertise in recognition of the impending danger, action to be taken for their prevention, correct dosing and adequate monitoring. The number of large follicles induced influences the chances of a multiple pregnancy, whereas large numbers of intermediate and small sized follicles contribute to the incidence of OHSS.

In general, overweight and obesity are serious impeding factors in the attaining of a live birth following ovulation induction and, for that matter, all other forms of treatment for infertility. Every attempt should be made to reduce the weight of overweight and frankly obese patients, by lifestyle changes involving dietary advice and exercise, before embarking on ovulation induction. Obesity not only negatively influences the chances of conception but also increases the prevalence of spontaneous miscarriage. This is especially relevant for women with infertility associated with PCOS as obesity exaggerates the deleterious effects of insulin resistance on fertility potential. A loss of just 5% or more of body weight is often enough to improve this situation.

Clomifene citrate

Indications

Clomifene citrate (CC) is the first-line treatment for women with absent or irregular ovulation associated with normal concentrations of endogenous estradiol and FSH (WHO Group 2, hypothalamic–pituitary dysfunction). A very large majority of these cases are associated with PCOS.

Mode of action

CC is an anti-oestrogenic compound closely resembling oestrogen which acts by blocking oestrogen receptors, particularly in the hypothalamus, thereby signalling a lack of circulating oestrogens and inducing a change in the pulsatile release of GnRH. This induces a discharge of FSH from the anterior pituitary and is often enough to reset the cycle of events leading to ovulation into motion.

Dose

CC (50mg tablets) is given orally in a dose of 50–150mg/day for 5 days from day 2, 3, 4 or 5 of a spontaneous or induced bleeding. The starting day of treatment does not seem to influence the results. The recommended dose for the first cycle of treatment is 50mg/day. If ovulation is achieved, there is no need to increase the dose in subsequent cycles. If there is no response, i.e. no evidence of ovulation, the dose may be increased in increments of 50mg in subsequent cycles until ovulation is achieved. An ovulatory response is reportedly achieved by 46% on 50mg/day, a further 21% respond to 100mg and another 8% to 150mg. Doses >150mg/day do not seem to confer any significant increase in either ovulation or pregnancy rates.

Results

Ovulation rate 75%, pregnancy rate 35%, live birth rate 28–30%, miscarriage rate 20%, twin pregnancy rate 8–13%, singleton live birth rate 22%. 'Clomifene failure' may be due to a failure to respond with ovulation to maximal doses (clomifene resistance) or a failure to conceive following six ovulatory cycles.

Factors affecting results

Clomifene resistance is more likely to occur in patients who are obese, insulin resistant and hyperandrogenic. A failure to conceive despite achieving ovulation may be due to the anti-oestrogen effects of CC; suppression of cervical mucous and/or suppression of endometrial development (<7mm thickness at mid-cycle). These effects are idiosyncratic, occur in ~15% of patients receiving CC, recur in repeated cycles, and are not dose dependent nor improved by adding oestrogen therapy. IUI can overcome suppression of the cervical mucous, but endometrial suppression should preclude further attempts at treatment with CC, and low-dose FSH or lapararoscopic ovarian drilling (LOD) may be offered. Persistently high serum concentrations of LH are also thought to reduce the chances of pregnancy.

Duration of treatment

75% of the pregnancies induced by CC occur in the first three cycles of treatment. Best practice is not to exceed 6 months or in some cases 12 months of treatment. There is little advantage to be gained by employing a dose of >150mg/day if this fails to produce ovulation. In this case, metformin added to CC, low-dose gonadotrophins or LOD may be offered. If six ovulatory cycles fail to yield a pregnancy, IUI is usually employed in addition to CC.

Monitoring

CC is often administered without any monitoring of the treatment cycle. This is not good practice as it is important to know whether ovulation has been achieved and whether endometrial development is normal. A vaginal ultrasound examination on day 12–14 of a treatment cycle should suffice as the number and size of developing follicles and endometrial thickness can be visualized easily. Knowledge of the response to CC regarding follicular and endometrial development may save many months of superfluous treatment with an insufficient dose or in the presence of endometrial suppression.

Adjuvants for treatment with CC

An ovulation-triggering dose of hCG (5000–10 000IU) when a follicle of 19–24mm is demonstrated is only theoretically warranted when ovulation is not forthcoming in the presence of a leading follicle of this size due to the absence of an LH surge. However, although the routine administration of hCG at mid-cycle seems to add little to the improvement of pregnancy rates, it is useful to aid the timing of IUI or intercourse. Dexamethasone (0.5mg daily at night) as an addition to CC treatment is probably best reserved for women who have evidence of an adrenal source of hyperandrogenism such as late-onset congenital adrenal hyperplasia. The possible pretreatment or addition of metformin to treatment with CC is dealt with below.

Side-effects

Adverse effects of clomifene are not common but include hot flushes, ovarian hyperstimulation, abdominal distension and visual disturbances.

Aromatase inhibitors

Although widely used for the treatment of postmenopausal women with advanced breast cancer, the use of aromatase inhibitors for induction of ovulation is still experimental and has not yet been fully sanctioned by the international community due to conflicting evidence regarding possible teratogenicity. The use of aromatase inhibitors for ovulation induction is briefly described here as, pending reassuring further data on the outcome of pregnancies, it is believed that their use for ovulation induction has some advantages over CC as first-line treatment for WHO Group 2 anovulatory women.

- Aromatase inhibitors are potent suppressors of oestrogen synthesis, blocking the action of the enzyme aromatase which converts androgens to oestrogens, temporarily releasing the hypothalamus from the negative feedback effect of oestrogen, so inducing an increased discharge of FSH.
- In contrast to CC, aromatase inhibitors have no effect on oestrogen receptors and therefore no deleterious effect on cervical mucus, endometrium and the hypothalamic negative feedback mechanism. The half-life of the aromatase inhibitors is ~2 days, much shorter than that of CC.
- Preliminary, small trials have demonstrated the theoretical advantages compared with CC, the lack of an anti-oestrogen effect on endometrium and less multiple follicle development, while being equally efficient as regards induction of ovulation. Large RCTs are awaited to confirm these preliminary results.

Metformin

Metformin is being prescribed to reduce insulin and androgen concentrations and treat anovulation associated with PCOS. Metformin is an oral biguanide, well established for the treatment of hyperglycaemia, that does not cause hypoglycaemia in normoglycaemic subjects. Although there is some conflicting evidence regarding the usefulness of metformin and despite the fact that it is not currently licensed for the management of PCOS, it is being widely prescribed.

Indications

For restoration of ovulation for women with PCOS, metformin may be given alone or as pretreatment and co-treatment with CC. Proof of insulin resistance is not a prerequisite for treatment as, first, this is difficult to assess accurately and, secondly, it does seem to predict the success of treatment.

Mode of action

Metformin is an insulin sensitizer which reduces insulin resistance and insulin secretion, followed by a reduction of ovarian androgen production. A direct action of metformin on ovarian theca cells also reduces androgen production.

Dose

Metformin is taken orally in doses of 1500–2500mg daily.

Side-effects

About 15–20% of patients may suffer gastrointestinal side-effects, some of which may be lessened by a graduated starting dose.

Metformin alone

Metformin is capable of improving menstrual frequency and restoring ovulation in patients who have oligo/anovulation and PCOS, although less effectively than clomiphene alone. However, for obese patients (BMI >30), metformin (1700mg/day) was no better than placebo in improving menstrual function, whereas weight loss was effective in this respect. Most studies have shown no increase or a modest increase only in pregnancy rates.

Metformin + CC

Some initial collected reports suggested that the combination of pretreatment and co-treatment of metformin with CC is significantly more successful in inducing ovulation and pregnancy compared with the use of metformin alone or CC alone. However, in previously untreated women with PCOS, no superiority of the combination of CC and metformin rather than CC alone was demonstrated in a large multicentre study from The Netherlands nor in a large American study that also demonstrated no superiority of the combination over metformin alone. However, metformin added to CC therapy in CC-resistant patients and CC administered to those who failed to ovulate on metformin alone will achieve ovulation and pregnancy in some women, and may be tried before turning to the more costly FSH therapy.

Metformin in IVF

Two well controlled studies have shown a considerable superiority in pregnancy rates in non-obese women with PCOS, compared with placebo, when metformin was started either 6 weeks before or at the start of a GnRH agonist long protocol.

Metformin in pregnancy

Metformin seems to be safe when continued into pregnancy, as no increase in congenital abnormalities, teratogenicity or adverse effects on infant development have been recorded. There is conflicting evidence regarding the ability of metformin to reduce the high miscarriage rate usually occurring in PCOS patients to levels seen in the normal population. Whether metformin should be continued into the pregnancy is still disputed. When taken throughout pregnancy, metformin may reduce the prevalence of gestational diabetes, macrosomia and pre-eclampsia in women with PCOS.

Pulsatile gonadotrophin-releasing hormone (Gonadorelin)

Pulsatile GnRH therapy is the classical treatment of anovulation associated with hypogonadotrophic hypogonadism (WHO Group 2) and can be regarded as pure replacement therapy to restore the function of the anterior pituitary in discharging FSH and LH. It can be used as an alternative to gonadotrophin therapy with both FSH and LH activity.

- GnRH is administered through an infusion pump, very similar to an insulin pump, either s.c. or i.v.
- The dose is a bolus of 15–20 micrograms s.c. or 5–10 micrograms i.v. every 60–90min. Very occasionally, thrombophlebitis is experienced at the site of the indwelling catheter using the i.v. route.
- Pulsatile GnRH is very effective treatment for idiopathic hypogonadotrophic hypogonadism, Kallmann's syndrome and low weight-related amenorrhea, producing pregnancy rates well in excess of 80%.
- Following ovulation, the pump must be continued into the luteal phase. If stopped following ovulation, then luteal phase support is required.
- For the treatment of WHO Group 1 anovulation, compared with gonadotrophin treatment, the GnRH has the advantage of producing a monofollicular ovulation in the vast majority of cycles and a consequent low rate of multiple pregnancy. The disadvantage of pulsatile GnRH therapy is the inconvenience of wearing the pump and accoutrements, and this has limited patient acceptability.

Gonadotrophins

Gonadotrophin preparations containing FSH provide an exogenous source for the direct stimulus of follicular development in anovulatory women. hCG mimics the action of the LH surge and is used to trigger ovulation once a stimulated follicle(s) has reached a stage of development when ovulation can be induced. The aim of ovulation induction with gonadotrophins is to produce, ideally, one ovulatory follicle, so avoiding the complications of multiple follicular development, OHSS and multiple pregnancies.

FSH-containing preparations

These preparations may be derived from human menopausal urine from which either FSH or FSH + LH are extracted and purified, or from the use of recombinant DNA technology to produce recombinant human FSH. Large RCTs and meta-analyses comparing the use of urinary-derived and recombinant preparations for ovulation induction have shown no significant differences regarding ovulation and pregnancy rates, miscarriage, hyperstimulation or multiple pregnancy rates. Technically, in comparison with urinary preparations, recombinant FSH is purer, containing less unwanted protein and other contaminants. As far as the outcome of gonadotrophin ovulation induction therapy is concerned, no clear clinical superiority has been demonstrated between preparations containing LH (hMG) and those containing FSH alone. Only for women with hypogonadotrophic hypogonadism is LH an essential component to ensure efficient and successful ovulation induction.

Delivery systems

Both recombinant FSH preparations (follitropin α and follitropin β) are now available as ready-to-use preparations in a pen injection device which comes either preloaded containing 300, 450 or 900IU (follitropin α, Gonal-F®, Serono) or in cartridges for loading containing 300, 600 or 900IU recombinant FSH (follitropin β, Puregon®, Organon). With pen devices, the FSH dose can be accurately titrated and individualized for each patient for s.c. injection, and is more user-friendly.

Indications

For ovulation induction, gonadotrophin therapy is indicated for hypogonadotrophic hypogonadism (WHO Group I) if preferred to pulsatile GnRH therapy. For women with hypogonadotrophic hypogonadism, it is essential to use an LH-containing preparation or to add recombinant LH to FSH in order to ensure efficient ovulation induction. More commonly, gonadotrophins are employed for those with WHO Group II anovulation who either did not respond to CC or failed to conceive following six ovulatory cycles on CC.

Treatment protocol

Conventional, regular protocol

Gonadotrophin treatment is started on day 2–5 of menstruation, natural or induced, when the ovary is quiescent and the endometrium thin. Using a regular, conventional protocol, the initial dose in the first cycle of treatment has usually been one ampoule a day of hMG (75IU FSH + 75IU LH) or 75–100IU of FSH with incremental dose rises of one ampoule of hMG or 50–75IU of FSH every 5–7 days if an inadequate response (no follicle >9mm) is recorded on ultrasound examination. Ovulation is triggered with a single i.m. injection of 5000–10 000IU of hCG when 1–3 follicles reach a diameter of at least 17mm. The starting dose in subsequent cycles could be adjusted according to the response in the previous cycle. The conventional protocol has been largely abandoned, certainly for women with Group II anovulation, as it produced multiple pregnancy rates of 34% and severe OHSS in 4.6%. As these figures are unacceptable today, a chronic low-dose protocol has been devised and applied.

Low-dose step-up protocol

The aim of the chronic low-dose step-up protocol is to obtain the ovulation of a single follicle. Unlike the conventional protocol, the low-dose protocol employs a dose of gonadotrophin that is not supra-physiological but reaches the threshold for a follicular response without exceeding it, thereby producing monofollicular rather than multifollicular ovulation. This practically eliminates the occurrence of OHSS and reduces multiple pregnancies to an acceptable rate. The chronic low-dose regimen (illustrated in Fig. 14.1) employs a small starting dose in the first cycle of treatment of 50–75IU of FSH which remains unchanged for 14 days. If this does not produce the criteria for hCG administration, a small incremental dose rise of 25–37.5IU is used every 7 days until follicular development is initiated. The dose that initiates follicular development (at least one follicle >10mm) is continued until the criteria for giving hCG are attained. hCG should not be given if ≥3 follicles >16mm diameter are seen. Using a starting dose of 75IU FSH ensures that ~90% of women will not require any dose adjustment, whereas starting with 50IU of FSH requires a dose adjustment in ~50% of women.

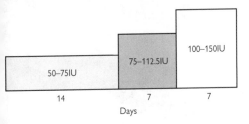

Fig. 14.1 The chronic low-dose step-up regimen for the administration of gonadotrophin.

Step-down protocol

On the basis of physiological principles concerning concentrations of FSH in a natural ovulatory cycle, a step-down protocol has been suggested starting with 150IU of FSH for 5 days, raising the dose by 37.5IU every 3 days if necessary, until a follicle of 10mm is obtained (Fig. 14.2). The daily dose is then reduced by 37.5IU every 3 days until the criteria for giving hCG are reached. However, although pregnancy rates are similar and FSH is given for a shorter duration with step-down, the low-dose step-up has a lower rate of overstimulation, double the rate of monofollicular ovulation and a higher ovulation rate, and is, therefore, preferred by most.

Monitoring

The timing of a possible increase in dose and the timing of hCG administration are the essence of efficient ovulation induction and the avoidance of OHSS and multiple pregnancies with gonadotrophin therapy. Accurate monitoring of follicular development by transvaginal ultrasound examination of the ovaries and endometrial thickness is the key factor. Most units also estimate serum estradiol and progesterone concentrations on the same day as the ultrasound examination, but some reserve these examinations only for women at high risk for OHSS. Using a conventional protocol, the first examination is usually performed on day 6 of stimulation, and with a low-dose protocol on day 8. Once an emerging follicle of ≥10mm diameter is seen, the daily effective dose used to achieve this should not be changed and further examinations performed every 2–3 days following. As a rough rule of thumb, an emerging leading follicle will grow at a rate of 2mm/day on the daily effective dose. The criteria for administering hCG in a dose of 5000–10 000IU are 1–2 follicles of ≥17mm. If hCG is given when >2 follicles of this size are attained, the risk of a multiple pregnancy is increased considerably and hCG should be withheld.

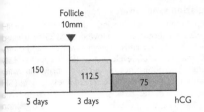

Fig. 14.2 The step-down protocol.

Ovarian hyperstimulation syndrome

OHSS is a serious complication of ovulation induction caused by over-stimulating the ovaries with gonadotrophins followed by hCG to trigger ovulation. It is an iatrogenic condition that is largely preventable and often foreseeable. Women at greatest risk of developing OHSS are young, lean and have polycystic ovaries. The occurrence of OHSS in a previous cycle is also a predisposing factor which should induce watchfulness.

Prevention of OHSS

- If hCG is withheld, OHSS will not occur.
- For patients with the above risk factors, a small starting dose and small incremental dose rises if needed in a chronic low-dose protocol will prevent OHSS.
- If the danger of OHSS looks imminent during ovulation stimulation (a large number of developing follicles, rapidly rising estradiol concentrations, very high estradiol concentrations >1500pg/mL or 5500pmol/mL), hCG should be withheld. It is better to 'lose' a cycle than take the risk of severe OHSS. Alternatively, coasting may be employed by withdrawing gonadotrophin therapy and checking the number and size of follicles and estradiol concentrations daily thereafter until hCG can safely be given when coasting has caused a regression in the number of follicles and a decrease in estradiol concentrations. Coasting has only proved to be effective if the interval between stopping gonadotrophins and giving hCG does not exceed 3 days.
- A less popular recourse for action if overstimulation occurs during ovulation induction entails follicle puncture, oocyte retrieval and IVF, so-called rescue IVF.
- Giving one injection of a GnRH agonist to trigger a release of endogenous LH in place of hCG has met with some success in ovulation induction facing possible OHSS. The shorter half-life of a GnRH agonist compared with hCG is thought to be the important difference between the two. For a similar reason, recombinant LH can be employed instead of hCG.

Prevention of multiple pregnancies

During ovulation induction, the risk of a multiple pregnancy increases when hCG is given when >2 large follicles have developed. The hCG injection should be withheld in this situation. Using a strict chronic low-dose protocol, this should be a rare occurrence.

Results

Using a conventional protocol for WHO Group I and Group II anovulation, a collection of results published in 1990 revealed a pregnancy rate of 46% but a multiple pregnancy rate of 34% and a prevalence of 4.6% of severe OHSS. Following the inception of a chronic low-dose protocol, while the pregnancy rate is similar, multiple pregnancy occurs in <6%, and OHSS has been virtually eliminated (Table 14.1).

Table 14.1 Results of treatment with chronic low-dose gonadotrophin

No. of patients	841
No. of cycles	1556
Pregnancies (% patients)	320 (38%)
Fecundity/cycle	20%
Uniovulation	70%
OHSS	0.14%
Multiple pregnancies	5.7%

Laparoscopic ovarian drilling (LOD)

The original treatment of PCOS instigated by Stein and Leventhal was bilateral wedge resection of the ovaries. Although producing restoration of ovulation in a high proportion of women and inducing pregnancy, it was abandoned due to a high prevalence of pelvic adhesion formation. The principle of operational treatment (presumably a reduction in ovarian mass) has been revived but by way of LOD.

• On laparoscopy, 4–10 punctures with a depth of 2–4mm are made in the cortex of each ovary. Fewer than four punctures are ineffective and >10 create too much damage to the ovary. Using bipolar or unipolar electrocautery, 40W for 4s for each puncture is a good rule of thumb. Laser can also be used, but electrocautery is reported to produce better results with less adhesion formation.

• An ovulation rate of 84% and a pregnancy rate of 56% were experienced within 1yr of LOD in the first collection of reports. A single-centre study of long-term follow-up revealed that 49% conceived spontaneously within a year and a further 38% conceived 1–9yrs after LOD. The cumulative conception rate after 30 months was 75%. If no ovulation results within 2–3 months of LOD, the administration of CC will induce ovulation in many who were previously resistant to CC and, if this is not successful, a low-dose FSH protocol can be applied. The addition of CC or FSH following drilling considerably increases pregnancy rates.

• Women with PCOS of normal weight and with high LH concentrations are those most likely to ovulate and conceive following treatment by LOD.

• The advantage of LOD for ovulation induction in women with PCOS is that, almost invariably, it will produce a monofollicular ovulation and therefore a very low rate of multiple pregnancies and no OHSS. In addition, the miscarriage rate following LOD (14%) is lower than that usually experienced with other forms of ovulation induction for PCOS.

Further reading

Hamilton-Fairly O,and Frank S. Common problems in induction of ovulation. Balliere's Clinical Obstetrics and Gynaecology 1990; **4**: 609–625.

Kousta E, White DM, Franks S.Modern use of clomiphene citrate in induction of ovulation. *Hum Reprod Update* 1997; **3**: 359–365.

Moll E, Bossuyt PM, Korevaar JC, Lambalk CB, van der Veen F. Effect of clomiphene citrate plus metformin and clomiphene citrate plus placebo on induction of ovulation in women with newly diagnosed polycystic ovary syndrome: a randomized double blind clinical trial. *BMJ* 2006; **332**: 1485.

Tubal and uterine disorders

Introduction

Normal conception requires a fertile sperm and egg to come together and a receptive endometrium to allow the resulting embryo to implant. Tubal damage underlies infertility in ~15% of couples. In some of these couples, it may be that the women has previously undergone a tubal sterilization procedure for conception but wish to have this reversed. Whereas tubal occlusion or damage is a relatively clear-cut cause of infertility, the presence of uterine fibroids is less absolute as an explanation for their infertility. This is also the cause for intra-uterine adhesion and congenital abnormalities of the uterus.

Tubal disorders

Any damage to the fallopian tube can prevent the sperm from reaching the oocyte or the embryo from reaching the uterine cavity, leading to infertility and tubal ectopic pregnancy. The fallopian tube is more than a simple 'tube'. It has cilia that assist in transport, it facilitates capacitation of the sperm, and fertilization and the early development of the zygote and embryo. Therefore, the fallopian tube may maintain its patency but lose the ability to promote these other functions.

Anatomy

The fallopian tubes are seromuscular paired tubular organs that run medially from the ovaries to the cornua of the uterus. The fallopian tubes are situated toward the upper margins of the broad ligament. The tubes connect the endometrial cavity in the uterus with the peritoneal cavity toward the ovaries on each side. The tubes average 10cm in length (range, 7–14cm). The tubes can be divided into four parts (proximally at the endometrial cavity to their distal portion near the ovary):

- The intramural or interstitial portion (from the endometrial cavity, through the uterine wall, and to the uterine cornua).
- The isthmus (the proximal third of the fallopian tubes outside the uterine wall).
- The ampulla (the distal two-thirds of the fallopian tubes outside the uterine wall).
- The infundibulum, the funnel-shaped opening to the peritoneal cavity.

The fimbria are finger-like extensions from the margins of the infundibulum toward the ovaries on each side. The intraluminal diameter varies and increases from 0.1mm in the intramural portion to 1cm in the ampullary portion of the tubes. The fallopian tubes receive their blood supply from the tubal branches of the uterine arteries and from small branches of the ovarian arteries. The fallopian tubes receive sensory, autonomic and vasomotor nerve fibres from the ovarian and inferior hypogastric plexi.

Pathophysiology

The main causes of tubal disease are either pelvic inflammatory disease (PID) or iatrogenic causes. PID commonly causes tubal blockage, either proximally at the site of insertion into the uterus or distally at the fimbrial end. Less commonly, a midtubal segment may become occluded. Blockage at two points results in a hydrosalpinx because the continued secretions of the tubal mucosa have no drainage into the peritoneal or uterine cavities. As the hydrosalpinx enlarges, the tubal muscularis thins. The secretory and ciliary properties of the endosalpinx are eventually disrupted. The probability of pregnancy after repair of hydrosalpinges with a diameter of >3cm is very poor.

The pathophysiology after tubal sterilization depends on the method used. The method used most in the UK is Filchie clips which cause the least 'damage' to the fallopian tube and are therefore easily reversed. Electrocautery of a segment or segments of the fallopian tube occludes the lumen and causes more damage to the surrounding tissues than placement of a ring or a clip over the mid portion of the tube or surgical interruption of the tube. Increasing the amount of damage to the fallopian tube may increase the success of the sterilization procedure, but it decreases the chance of achieving subsequent successful reconstruction. The length of a tube after a reconstructive procedure correlates with success in terms of achieving pregnancy. Patients with tubes >5cm after reconstruction have better outcomes than patients whose tubes measure ≤3cm.

Any inflammatory condition in the pelvis, such as endometriosis or the sequelae of pelvic or abdominal surgery, may cause adhesions, tubal blockage or injury to the tubal mucosa and/or muscularis, resulting in tubal damage and dysfunction. In some women, cornual polyps may develop in the fallopian tube, causing a blockage that may be reversible by resection of the polyp.

Salpingitis isthmica nodosa

Proximal tubal disease can also be caused by salpingitis isthmica nodosa. It is commonly diagnosed when firm nodules are found on the fallopian tubes. The diagnosis is confirmed by histopathology. The hallmark of salpingitis isthmica nodosa is the presence of diverticula or outpouchings of the tubal epithelium, which are surrounded by hypertrophied smooth muscle. The diagnosis can only be confirmed by histology. It can be suspected by hysterosalpingography if proximal obstruction is present or by a stippled appearance indicating contrast medium in the diverticular projections. It is commonly bilateral and often found in fertile women. The cause of salpingitis isthmica nodosa is not known. Salpingitis isthmica nodosa is found in 0.6–11% of healthy fertile women and is almost always bilateral.

Surgery to the fallopian tube

Any surgery to the fallopian tube that is designed to restore or improve fertility should use microsurgical techniques. These technique are more commonly used at open surgery but are increasingly being performed through endoscopic surgery. Microsurgical technique is a delicate surgical style that emphasizes the use of magnification, fine atraumatic instrumentation, microsuturing, continuous irrigation to prevent desiccation, and pinpoint haemostasis. The goals are to remove pathology, restore normal anatomy and regain function with minimal damage to adjacent normal tissue. This is achieved by minimizing inflammation and preventing adhesion formation.

Intramural/interstitial obstruction

This is one of the more challenging surgeries to perform as it often involves tubal re-implantation after the resection of cornual polyps. In some cases patency can be restored by hysteroscopic or radiological cannulation. The tubal ostia are visualized in the endometrial cavity with the hysteroscope or under radiological control. A small wire is inserted through the os into the intramural portion of the tube, and a small catheter is threaded over the wire. Patency can be confirmed when dye introduced through the small catheter in the intramural portion of the tube is visualized extruding through the fimbria via laparoscopy or radiologically.

Isthmic and midportion occlusion (including reversal of sterilization)

Isthmic occlusion can be repaired by performing an isthmic–cornual or an isthmic–isthmic anastomosis as appropriate. The damaged portion of the tube is transected perpendicular to the axis of the tube. The occluded portion of the tube is resected 2mm at a time, initially proximally and subsequently distally, until the tubal lumen is visualized. Proximal patency is confirmed using retrograde methylene blue through a cannula in the uterine cavity. Distal patency is confirmed by threading a piece of thin suture material from the fimbrial end toward the area of anastomosis.

An anchoring suture is placed in the proximal and distal mesosalpinx (isthmic–isthmic repair) or from the cornu proximally to the mesosalpinx distally (cornual–isthmic repair) to bring the two portions of the tube being reanastomosed in proximity. Four interrupted sutures are placed at the 12-, 3-, 6- and 9-o'clock positions, parallel to the axis of the tube, first within the muscularis (using a 8.0 non-absorbable suture, e.g. prolene) and subsequently on the serosa (6.0 prolene), to bring together the proximal and distal portions of the tube.

For reversal of sterilization, depending on the age, pregnancy rates should be in the order of 80% in the first year.[1]

---

[1] Boeckx W, Gordts S, Buysse K, Brosens I. Reversibility after female sterilization. *Br J Obstet Gynaecol* 1986; **93**: 839–842.

Occlusion of the distal portion of the fallopian tube

This usually involves a fimbroplasty. Proximal patency of the tube should be confirmed with a preoperative hysterosalpingogram. Filling the fallopian tube with dilute dye at the time of surgery (via a cannula in the uterine cavity) facilitates identification of the entrance point in the distal, peritoneal surface of the tube that opens into the tubal lumen. The entrance point, which should be relatively avascular, is then opened using scissors, needle point diathermy or laser. The fimbria are then retracted using either sutures or thermal damage to the peritoneal surface of the tube proximal to the fimbria.

Results of surgery

A case series study reported that 27, 47 and 53% of women with proximal tubal blockage who had microsurgical tubocornual anastomosis achieved a live birth within 1, 2 and 3.5 years of surgery, respectively. A review of nine other case series studies reported that ~50% of women with proximal tubal blockage who had microsurgical tubocornual anastomosis achieved a term pregnancy, but it did not specify the time period upon which this figure was based. Surgery is more effective in women with milder pelvic disease (stage I, 67%, stage, II 41%; stage III, 12%; and stage, IV 0%).

Uterine disorders

Submucous leiomyomata, congenital uterine abnormalities, endometrial polyps and intra-uterine adhesions are all potential causes of infertility. The presence of a fibroid that distorts the fallopian tubes will lead to tubal infertility. Distortion of the uterine cavity, by a fibroid, a septum or a congenitally mis-shaped uterus, can lead to implantation failure and/or recurrent miscarriage. Recent evidence has also suggested that intramural fibroids may also inhibit implantation to a certain degree. It is not yet known, however, if removal of these intramural fibroids with result in an increased fertility level.

Excessive uterine curettage, e.g. after a miscarriage, especially in the presence of infection, can lead to the distortion of the strata basalis endometrium. Intra-uterine scarification and synechiae develop as a result, and this is known as Asherman's syndrome.

Uterine fibroids

The incidence of myoma in women with infertility without any other cause for their infertility is estimated to be ~2%.

Submuscosal fibroids may be removed hysteroscopically, with intramural and subserosal fibroids being removed either at open surgery or, if <9cm in size, laparoscopically.

Microsurgical techniques as described above should be used and, if available, anti-adhesion devices used following surgery for intramural and subserosal fibroids.

Medical and surgical management of endometriosis

Introduction

Endometriosis is characterized by the presence of endometrial tissue (glandular and stromal tissue) in areas outside the uterus. It has been considered for decades to be the result of the implantation of retrograde menstruated endometrial cells (Sampson's theory), or as metaplasia induced by menstrual debris or as lymphatic spread. It occurs most frequently in the pelvic organs and peritoneum, and is prevalent in 2.5–3.3% of women of reproductive age. Endometriosis is a surgical diagnosis. In a hospital-based population, however, the prevalence of endometriosis will vary depending on the type of the population being studied, e.g. it is seen more frequently among women being investigated for infertility (21%) than among those undergoing sterilization (6%). The incidence of endometriosis among those women being investigated for chronic abdominal pain is 15%, while among those undergoing abdominal hysterectomy, it can be as high as 25%.

Examination and investigations

The symptoms associated with endometriosis, principally dysmenorrhoea, dyspareunia and pelvic pain, are common. Establishing the diagnosis can be difficult because the presentation is so variable and there is considerable overlap with other conditions such as irritable bowel syndrome and PID. As a result, there is often delay between symptom onset and surgical diagnosis.

Endometriosis may present with any combination of the following: secondary dysmenorrhoea, deep dyspareunia, pelvic pain, infertility or a pelvic mass. However, the predictive value of any one symptom or set of symptoms remains uncertain. Furthermore, endometriosis is often found coincidentally in asymptomatic women.

Laparoscopy is still regarded for the moment as the 'gold standard' diagnostic test looking for evidence of all types and stages of endometriosis. However, diagnostic laparoscopy is associated with 0.06% risk of major complications (e.g. bowel perforation), whilst this risk is increased to 1.3% in operative laparoscopy.

The use of transvaginal ultrasound may be helpful in diagnosis, particularly to detect ovarian endometriomas. A systematic review on the accuracy of ultrasound identified seven relevant studies, all using transvaginal scanning (TVS) to diagnose endometriomas. The positive likelihood ratios ranged from 7.6 to 29.8, and the negative likelihood ratios ranged from 0.12 to 0.4. TVS therefore appears to be a useful test both to make and to exclude the diagnosis of an ovarian endometrioma. MRI may be a useful non-invasive tool in the diagnosis of endometriosis, particularly deep endometriosis. While it has limitations in the visualization of the smallest endometriotic implants and adhesions, it has the ability to characterize the lesions and to study extraperitoneal locations and the contents of pelvic masses.

Serum CA-125 testing has limited value as a screening test for endometriosis. The performance of CA-125 measurement has been assessed in a meta-analysis: 23 studies have investigated serum CA-125 levels in women with surgically confirmed endometriosis. The test's performance in diagnosing all disease stages was limited: the estimated sensitivity was only 28% for a specificity of 90% (corresponding likelihood ratio of a raised level was 2.8). The test's performance for moderate to severe endometriosis was better: for a specificity of 89%, the sensitivity was 47% (corresponding likelihood ratio of a raised level was 4.3). The routine use of serum CA-125 testing, particularly in subfertile patients, may therefore be justified to identify a subgroup of women who are likely to benefit from early laparoscopy. Thus CA-125 has limited value as a screening test as well as a diagnostic test. It may, however, serve as a useful marker for monitoring the effect of treatment once the diagnosis of endometriosis has been established, but again its use has not been evaluated systematically.

The choice of treatment will depend upon the woman's age, her fertility plans, previous treatment, the nature and severity of the symptoms, and the location and severity of disease.

Endometriosis-associated infertility

Arguments that support the hypothesis of a strong association, possibly a causal relationship, between the presence of endometriosis and subfertility include:

- An increased prevalence of endometriosis in subfertile women when compared with women of proven fertility.
- A trend towards a reduced monthly fecundity rate in infertile women with minimal to mild endometriosis when compared with women with unexplained infertility.
- A dose–effect relationship: a negative correlation between the revised American Fertility Society (AFS) stage of endometriosis and the monthly fecundity rate and crude pregnancy rate.
- A reduced number of oocytes, fertilization rate, implantation rate per embryo and pregnancy rate after IVF in women with moderate to severe endometriosis when compared with women with a normal pelvis.
- An increased monthly fecundity rate and cumulative pregnancy rate after surgical removal of minimal to mild endometriosis.

Surgical treatment of endometriosis

In most women with endometriosis, preservation of reproductive function is desirable. Therefore, the least invasive and least expensive approach that is effective should be used. The goal of surgery is to excise, coagulate or evaporate all visible endometriotic peritoneal lesions, endometriotic ovarian cysts, deep rectovaginal endometriosis and associated adhesions, and to restore normal anatomy. Surgery should be performed by laparoscopy as this affords the magnification and detail required to remove all lesions, as well as having the minimal invasive benefits over laparotomy. For more severe disease, referral to a centre specializing in endometriosis surgery may be required

Cystic ovarian endometriosis

The physiopathology of cystic endometriosis is not entirely understood. It is postulated that many cases of cystic ovarian endometriosis may originate from invagination of superficial implants. The management of ovarian cystic endometriosis (endometriomas) will depend to some extent on the size of the cyst. Small ovarian endometriomata (<3cm diameter) can be aspirated and irrigated; their interior wall can be vaporized to destroy the mucosal lining of the cyst. Large (>3cm in diameter) ovarian endometriomata should be aspirated, followed by incision and removal of the cyst wall from the ovarian cortex. To prevent recurrence, the cyst wall of the endometrioma must be removed and normal ovarian tissue must be preserved (Table 16.1). In large endometrioma (>5cm), it may be beneficial to perform the cytectomy as a two-stage procedure. The first operation to fenestrate and drain the endometrioma is followed by 3 months of a GnH analogue to shrink the cyst, then followed by a further laparoscopy to remove the cyst (Fig. 16.1). In this way minimal damage may be done to the cortex of the ovary. The use of the combined oral contraceptive (COC) prior to surgery may help to avoid confusion or inadvertent surgery on a corpus luteum.

Table 16.1 Removal versus ablation

Recurrence after coagulation or laser	Recurrence after cystectomy
18.4%	6.4%

The results were from a systematic review of four comparative trials.
Common odds ratio: 3.09 (95% CI 1.78–5.36).
From Vercellini P, Chapron C, De Giorgi O, Consonni D, Frontino G, Crosignani PG. Coagulation or excision of ovarian endometriomas? *Am J Obstet Gynecol* 2003; **188**: 606–610.

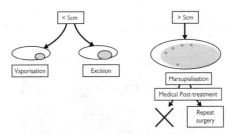

Fig. 16.1 Treatment of cystic ovarian endometriosis.

Deep rectovaginal and rectosigmoidal endometriosis

Endometriosis can infiltrate the surrounding tissues, resulting in a sclerotic and inflammatory reaction which can translate clinically into nodularity, bowel stenosis and ureteral obstruction. The most severe forms are rectovaginal endometriosis and endometriosis invading the rectum or the sigmoid. Three subtypes are described (Fig. 16.2).

- Type 1: large pelvic area of typical and sometimes some subtle endometriotic lesions surrounded by white sclerotic tissue.
- Type 2: characterized by retraction of the bowel. Clinically they are recognized by the obvious bowel retraction around a small typical lesion.
- Type 3: spherical endometriotic nodules in the rectovaginal septum. In their most typical manifestation these lesions are felt as painful nodularities in the rectovaginal septum.

Type 3 lesions are the most severe lesions, and they often spread laterally up and around the uterine artery, sometimes causing sclerosis around the ureter. Sclerosing endometriosis invading the sigmoid is similar to rectal endometriosis, but is situated 10cm above the rectovaginal septum. This is another form of deep endometriosis, which fortunately is a rare condition.

Surgery for deep endometriosis is unpredictably difficult, with the risk of a series of severe complications. Therefore, a preoperative ultrasound, contrast enema and i.v. pyelography are necessary in many cases, together with a full preoperative bowel preparation. Surgery should be carefully planned. This planning comprises preoperative ureter stenting if gross ureteric distortion or hydronephrosis is present, together with the eventual collaboration of a urologist to perform ureter re-anastomosis or repair, bladder suturing or ureter re-implantation. Preoperative planning often requires the collaboration of a colorectal surgeon, since surgery can unpredictably extend from a discoid excision with a muscularis defect, to a resection of the rectum or sigmoid wall necessitating a suture, to a large transmural nodule requiring a resection anastomosis if the defect is too large, or, in the case of a combined rectal and sigmoid nodule which cannot be sutured, a pouch anastomosis requiring mobilization of the left hemicolon.

The majority of women who have pain as a result of their endometriosis will also desire fertility. The result of fertility after surgery should therefore be considered.

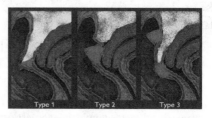

Fig. 16.2 Deep rectovaginal or sigmoidal endometriosis.

NICE Guidelines (2004)

The National Institute for Health and Clinical Excellence (NICE) recently reported on subfertility. Their conclusions regarding endometriosis were:

1. Women with minimal or mild endometriosis who undergo laparoscopy should be offered surgical ablation or resection of endometriosis plus laparoscopic adhesiolysis because this improves the chance of pregnancy.
2. Women with ovarian endometriomas should be offered laparoscopic cystectomy because this improves the chances of pregnancy.
3. Women with moderate or severe endometriosis should be offered surgical treatment because it improves the chances of pregnancy.
4. Postoperative medical treatment does not improve pregnancy rates in women with moderate to severe endometriosis and is not recommended.

Medical treatment

Because oestrogen is known to stimulate the growth of endometriosis hormonal therapy has been designed to suppress oestrogen synthesis, thereby inducing atrophy of ectopic endometrial implants or interrupting the cycle of stimulation and bleeding. Implants of endometriosis react to gonadal steroid hormones in a manner similar but not identical to normally stimulated ectopic endometrium. Ectopic endometrial tissue displays histological and biochemical differences from normal ectopic endometrium in characteristics such as glandular activity (proliferation, secretion), enzyme activity (17-α-hydroxysteroid dehydrogenase) and steroid (oestrogen, progestin and androgen) hormone receptor levels.

Oral contraceptive pill

The treatment of endometriosis with continuous low-dose monophasic combination contraceptives (one pill per day for 6–12 months) has been shown to be effective in reducing dysmenorrhoea and pelvic pain. In addition, the subsequent amenorrhoea induced by oral contraceptives could potentially reduce the amount of retrograde menstruation (one of the many risk factors proposed in the aetiology of endometriosis), decreasing the risk of disease progression. There is no convincing evidence that medical therapy with the COC offers definitive therapy. Instead, the endometrial implants survive the induced atrophy, with reactivation in most patients following termination of treatment.

There is no convincing evidence that cyclic use of combined oral contraceptives (COCs) provide prophylaxis against either the development or recurrence of endometriosis. Oestrogens in oral contraceptives potentially may stimulate the proliferation of endometriosis. The reduced menstrual bleeding that often occurs in women taking oral contraceptives may be beneficial to women with prolonged, frequent menstrual bleeding, which is a known risk factor for endometriosis

Progestins

Progestins may exert an anti-endometriotic effect by causing initial decidualization of endometrial tissue followed by atrophy. They can be considered as the first choice for the treatment of endometriosis because they are as effective in reducing AFS scores and pain as danazol or GnRH analogues, and have a lower cost and a lower incidence of side-effects than danazol or GnRH analogues. Medroxyprogesterone acetate (MPA) has been the most studied agent and is effective in relieving pain starting at a dose of 30mg/day and increasing the dose based on the clinical response and bleeding patterns. Side-effects of progestins include nausea, weight gain, fluid retention, and breakthrough bleeding due to hypo-oestrogenaemia. Depression and other mood disorders are a significant problem in ~1% of women taking these medications.

Local progesterone treatment of endometriosis-associated dysmenorrhoea with a levonorgestrel-releasing intra-uterine system (IUS; Mirena®, Organon Laboratories) during 12 months resulted in two studies in a significant reduction in dysmenorrhoea, pelvic pain and dyspareunia, a high degree of patient satisfaction and a significant reduction in volume of rectovaginal endometriotic nodules. Although the results are promising, none of these pilot studies included a control group. Further randomized evidence is needed before intra-uterine progesterone treatment can be introduced as a new drug effective in the suppression of endometriosis.

In the future, progesterone antagonists and progesterone receptor modulators may suppress endometriosis based on their anti-proliferative effects on the endometrium, without risk of hypo-oestrogenism or bone loss as after GnRH treatment.

Gonadotropin-releasing hormone agonists

GnRH agonists bind to pituitary GnRH receptors and stimulate LH and FSH synthesis and release. However, the agonists have a much longer biological half-life (3–8h) than endogenous GnRH (3.5min), resulting in the continuous exposure of GnRH receptors to GnRH agonist activity. This causes a loss of pituitary receptors and downregulation of GnRH activity, resulting in low FSH and LH levels. Consequently, ovarian steroid production is suppressed, providing a medically induced and reversible state of pseudomenopause. This results in atrophy of the ectopic endometrial tissue. The side-effects of GnRH agonist are a result of the hypo-oestrogenism caused, and include hot flashes, vaginal dryness, reduced libido and osteoporosis (6–8% loss in trabecular bone density after 6 months of therapy). To prevent these, 'add back' therapy in the form of HRT can be used.

Danazol

Pharmacological properties of danazol include suppression of GnRH, direct inhibition of steroidogenesis, increased metabolic clearance of estradiol and progesterone, direct antagonistic and agonistic interaction with endometrial androgen and progesterone receptors, and immunological attenuation of potentially adverse reproductive effects. The multiple effects of danazol produce a high-androgen, low-oestrogen environment that does not support the growth of endometriosis, and the amenorrhoea that is produced prevents new seeding of implants from the uterus into the peritoneal cavity. The significant adverse side-effects of danazol are related to its androgenic and hypo-oestrogenic properties. The most common side-effects include weight gain, fluid retention, acne, oily skin, hirsutism, hot flushes, atrophic vaginitis, reduced breast size, reduced libido, fatigue, nausea, muscle cramps and emotional instability. Deepening of the voice is another potential side-effect that is non-reversible.

Danazol is not more effective than other available medications to treat endometriosis, and is therefore not commonly used.

Aromatase inhibitors

Treatment of rats with induced endometriosis using the non-steroidal aromatase inhibitor fadrozole hydrochloride or YM511 resulted in dose-dependent volume reduction of the endometriosis transplants, but these products have so far not been used in published human studies.

Comparsion of different medical treatments for endometriosis

> *Combined oral contraceptive (COC) vs GnRH agonist (RCT = 1)*
>
> EE 20/DSG 150 as effective as goserelin for symptom relief.
>
> *Progestagens vs other medical therapy or placebo (RCTs = 4)*
>
> EE 35/CPA 27, EE 20/DSG 150, dydrogesterone and MPA as effective as goserelin or danazol for symptom relief.
>
> *Danazol (alone or as adjunctive therapy) vs placebo (RCTs = 4)*
>
> Danazol more effective than placebo in relieving symptoms and causing disease regression.
>
> *GnRH agonists vs other medical therapy or placebo (RCTs = 26)*
>
> GnRH agonists as effective as other active comparators (principally danazol) in relieving symptoms and causing disease regression.

Royal College of Obstetricians and Gynaecologists conclusion on medical therapy and endometriosis

'The choice between the combined oral contraceptive, progestagens, danazol and GnRH agonists depends principally upon their side-effect profiles because they relieve pain associated with endometriosis equally well' and that 'there is no role for medical therapy with hormonal drugs in the treatment of endometriosis associated infertility'.

Drug treatment	Side-effects
NSAIDs, e.g. mefenamic acid	Gastric irritation
Combined oral contraceptives	Nausea, migraines, increased risk of thromboembolism
Progestogens, e.g. norethisterone	Fluid retention, bloating and breast tenderness
Synthetic androgens, e.g. danazol	Androgenic, e.g. acne, weight gain
Gonadotrophin-releasing hormone agonists	Menopausal symptoms, osteoporosis (these can be countered by 'add back' therapy with HRT

Further reading and information

The endometriosis society: http://www.eshre.com/emc.asp

Mol BW, Bayram N, Lijmer JG, Wiegerinck MA, Bongers MY, Van der Veen F, Bossuyt PM. Fertil Steril. The performance of CA-125 measurement in the detection of endometriosis: a meta-analysis. 1998 Dec; **70**(6): 1101–8.

ESHRE guidelines for the diagnosis and treatment of endometrosis: http://guidelines. endometriosis.org/

McVeigh E, Koninckx PR. Surgery for advanced endometriosis. In: Bonnar J, ed. *Recent Advances in Obstetrics and Gynaecology 23*. London:Royal Society of Medicine Press Ltd.

Intra-uterine insemination

Introduction

- Intra-uterine insemination (IUI) involves the timed introduction of selected sperm into the uterine cavity.
- This is performed around the time of ovulation in unstimulated or stimulated cycles.
- The usual indications for IUI are mild male factor fertility problems or idiopathic (unexplained) infertility.

Methods

Three main methods are in use for the preparation of a fresh semen sample for IUI.
- Density gradient centrifugation.
- Swim-up.
- Washing in combination with centrifugation.

Of these, density gradient centrifugation is reported to be the most efficient.

Following sperm preparation, the sample is introduced in the peri-ovulatory period into the uterine cavity using a standard catheter designed for this purpose. One insemination per treatment cycle has been shown to be as effective as two inseminations per cycle given 24h apart.

Principle

IUI was originally suggested for the treatment of mild male factor infertility. The purpose of the laboratory treatment of the semen sample is to provide an 'improved' sample by selecting actively motile sperm in an increased density. This sample can then be safely inserted into the uterine cavity through the cervix, thus placing a bolus of concentrated motile sperm closer to the available egg(s).

Indications

- Mild male factor (sperm count <20 but >5 million/mL and/or progressive motility <50% but >20%) infertility and idiopathic (unexplained) infertility are the two main indications for IUI.
- The criteria for using IUI for the treatment of mild male factor infertility vary from clinic to clinic, but generally IUI is employed if the semen is of sufficient quality for there to be 1–5 million motile sperm available after sperm preparation. Less than 1 million motile sperm should indicate the use of IVF and ICSI rather than IUI.
- IUI is widely used for the empirical treatment of idiopathic infertility in both stimulated and unstimulated cycles. The combination of IUI with stimulated cycles, although improving pregnancy rates, is often accompanied by unacceptable multiple pregnancy rates. This suggests that the additional efficacy of stimulating the ovaries before IUI for unexplained infertility is due to multifollicular development, although correction of an undetected subtle defect in ovulatory function is also a possible contributory factor.

IUI for mild male factor infertility

- IUI is more successful than both timed intercourse and intracervical insemination in couples with mild male infertility, whether in stimulated or natural cycles.
- A systematic review of the literature revealed no significant difference between the results of IUI in stimulated and unstimulated cycles (pregnancy rates 13.7% vs 8.4% per cycle, respectively) for this indication.

IUI for unexplained infertility

- IUI with gonadotrophin stimulation for this indication has proved to be more effective than gonadotrophins alone.
- Stimulated cycles in combination with IUI are more effective than unstimulated cycles as regards pregnancy rates, but are often accompanied by unacceptable multiple pregnancy rates.
- IUI + hMG (pregnancy rate 18% per cycle) was found to be more effective than IUI + CC (6.7%) and IUI in a natural cycle (4%) in an analysis of 45 reports.
- Two large studies involving IUI in stimulated cycles, one from the USA employing an aggressive protocol starting with 150IU of FSH and one from the UK apparently employing a milder stimulation regime, illustrate the influence of gonadotrophin dosage on the multiple pregnancy rate. The American study reported 77 pregnancies including 22 multiples (3 sets of triplets and 2 quadruplets) whereas of the 126 pregnancies in the British study, just 14 were multiples (2 triplets and 1 set of quadruplets).
- In a Dutch study, a constant dose of 75IU FSH was used in the first cycle and hCG withheld if >3 follicles >17mm developed. If mono follicular development was seen in the first cycle, the dose for the next cycle was increased by 37.5IU. Live birth rates per monofollicular cycle were 7% compared with 10% when more than one follicle >13mm developed.
- A chronic low-dose step-up protocol of gonadotrophin stimulation for IUI with strict criteria for withholding hCG (given on mono- or bifollicular development only) is being examined in an attempt to reduce multiple pregnancy rates in IUI treatment without unduly compromising pregnancy rates. Results so far indicate that a pregnancy rate of 12–13% per cycle can be achieved. This type of ovarian stimulation may prove to be the compromise when balancing the low pregnancy rates of a natural cycle with the high multiple pregnancy rates of conventional gonadotrophin stimulation and IUI.
- The use of a GnRH antagonist in the stimulation protocol before IUI does not improve pregnancy rates.

Cost-effectiveness

For unexplained infertility, gonadotrophin-stimulated cycles for IUI produce the best pregnancy rates but the highest multiple pregnancy rates. When compared with IUI in unstimulated cycles, the price of medication and the possible need for neonatal treatment of prematurely delivered multiple pregnancies raise the question of cost-effectiveness. Should the price of gonadotrophin preparations be lowered (highly unlikely) or a low-dose gonadotrophin stimulation prove effective, cost-effectiveness would be less of an issue. As it is, some units have decided to sacrifice higher pregnancy rates and use purely natural cycles or resort to stimulated cycles after the failure of IUI in unstimulated cycles. These issues are not merely economic but also philosophical, e.g. what should be the cost of creating a human life? In this situation, each unit should adopt its own policy.

Conclusions

- IUI is a reasonably effective treatment for mild male factor and idiopathic infertility.
- It is generally reported that ovarian stimulation with gonadotrophins improves results for unexplained infertility when combined with IUI for this indication. This combination is superior to gonadotrophins alone or IUI alone.
- For the treatment of mild male factor infertility, gonadotrophin stimulation before IUI does not significantly improve results.
- The problem of unacceptable multiple pregnancy rates using gonadotrophin stimulation with IUI may be overcome by using a mild stimulation protocol and strict criteria for withholding hCG.

Further reading

Cohlen BJ, Vanderkerckhove P, te Velde ER, Habbema ID. Timed intercourse versus intra-uterine insemination with or without ovarian hyperstimulation for subfertility in men. *Cochrane Database Syst Rev* 2000; (2): CD000360.

Goverde AJ, McDonnell J, Vermeiden JP, Schats R, Rutten F, Schoemaker J. Intrauterine insemination or *in-vitro* fertilization in idiopathic sub-fertility and male subfertility: a randomised trial and cost-effectiveness analysis. *Lancet* 2000; **355**: 13–18.

In vitro fertilization and associated assisted conception techniques

Introduction

In vitro fertilization (IVF) refers to the extracorporeal fertilization of an oocyte. The term is, however, more loosely used to refer to the whole process of ovarian stimulation, oocyte retrieval, IVF and embryo transfer (ET). IVF-ET was initially developed to treat women with tubal infertility; it is now, however, an established treatment for a wide variety of infertility diagnoses including unexplained infertility. A number of factors should be considered for patient selection these include:

• Is there adequate ovarian reserve? An indication for this can be obtained from the age of the female and her early follicular (day 2–5) FSH level. As female age increases (>36yrs) and as FSH rises (>10IU/L) then ovarian response to exogenous FSH stimulation will decrease.

• Is there any underlying medical, surgical or psychological problems, e.g. severe renal disease or bowel adhesions secondary to Crohns' disease such that oocyte retrieval is not possible or safe?

• Is pregnancy safe for the woman and fetus? Are there any concerns over the welfare of any children born, e.g. history of domestic violence in the household?

Factors affecting the outcome of IVF

The single most important prognostic factor for successful IVF is the female age, as shown in Fig. 18.1.

Before IVF is commenced, the female should have her FSH level measured in the early follicular phase. This will give some indication as to the ovarian reserve and the success or otherwise of treatment.

The consumption of more than one unit of alcohol per day reduces the effectiveness of assisted reproduction procedures, including IVF treatment. It has also been shown that maternal and paternal smoking can have a similar adverse effect on the the success rates. An elveated body mass index (BMI) >30 will not only decrease the change of IVF working but will also increase the miscarriage rate of a subsequent pregnancy.

Recent studies have demonstrated that the presence of hydrosalpinges may decrease the implantation rate of embryos following IVF. RCTs have shown that the removal of these hydrosalpinges prior to IVF increases the success rate. The psychological effects of a salpingectomy must not be ignored, and restorative surgery (fimbroplasty) should also be considered.

The effect of stress on fertility and IVF has been and continues to be under study. To date, the evidence suggests that stress does not affect the outcome of IVF. The psychological welfare of the IVF couple, however, should be cared for in parallel to their physiological welfare. Counselling services should be available before, during and after this stressful intervention.

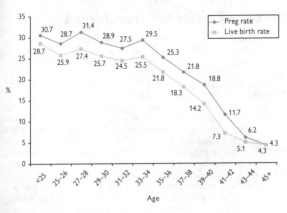

Fig. 18.1 IVF live birth rate by age.

Number of embryos transferred

The widespread use of assisted reproductive technologies has caused an exponential increase in the multiple pregnancy rates. Between 1980 and 1993, twin pregnancies increased by 25% and triplet and higher order pregnancies nearly tripled. In the USA the incidence of triplet and higher order pregnancies quadrupled from 1337 births in 1980 to 6737 births in 1997. These pregnancies are at significant risk of perinatal and maternal morbidity and mortality, with considerable medical, social and financial implications. Neonatal deaths are 7 times greater for twins and 23 times greater for triplets and higher order pregnancies than for singleton pregnancies. The stillbirth rate is 3 times greater for twins and >4 times greater for triplet and higher order pregnancies when compared with singletons. Mothers are at increased risk of pre-eclampsia, anaemia, ante- and post-partum haemorrhage and preterm labour, whilst fetuses are at increased risk of congenital malformation, intra-uterine growth restriction and complications of prematurity. Cerebral palsy is 5 times more common in twins and 17 times more common in triplets. The desire to increase the pregnancy rate through the transfer of increasing numbers of embryos must be balanced against this background. In the UK, the Human Fertilization and Embryology Authority (HFEA) regulations permit up to two embryos to be transferred in women under the age of 40 years old and three embryos in women over the age of 40 years.

Regulation of IVF

In the first 10 years following the birth of Louise Brown, there were no regulations in any country governing assisted reproduction techniques or research. Due to increasing pressure from within society, several countries now operate under laws and voluntary guidelines. A minority of countries such as Belgium, Finland, Greece, India and Portugal still have no laws or regulations. In the UK, the HFEA was established in 1990 following an Act of Parliament. This authority, which has statutory powers, licenses and inspects assisted conception units as well as regulating permissible areas of research involving human gametes and embryos. Through continued debate in society followed by licensing and inspection of IVF units, the HFEA can maintain assisted conception technology and techniques at an acceptable public level.

Procedures used during IVF

The IVF treatment cycle can be broken down into a number of different parts:
- Ovarian stimulation.
- Oocyte retrieval.
- *In vitro* fertilization.
- Embryo transfer.
- Luteal support.

Ovarian stimulation

In order to obtain a number of oocytes, exogenous stimulation of the ovaries is required. If this is done without 'control' of the hypothalamic–pituitary–ovarian axis, then premature luteinization and ovulation may occur. Attempts have been made to carry out 'natural' IVF cycles with no ovarian stimulation or pituitary modulation used. This method, however, leads to high cancellation rates due to a premature LH rise, and embryos are transferred in <50% of cycles, with an ongoing pregnancy rate <10% per cycle. There is also no control over the timing of oocyte retrieval as this needs to be performed 26–28h after detection of the endogenous LH surge. Therefore, this method is still relatively expensive as it requires monitoring, oocyte retrieval and laboratory work.

The basis of modern IVF is the transvaginal retrieval of mature oocytes from gonadotrophin-stimulated ovaries on the background of pituitary suppression.

Problems with premature LH rise led to the use of GnRH agonists and, more recently, GnRH antagonists. Initially GnRH agonists were started with ovarian stimulation ('flare' or short cycle), but more commonly now they are used for 2–3 weeks alone to achieve pituitary suppression ('long' cycle) followed by exogenous gonadotrophins for ovarian stimulation.

Types of agonist

Endogenous GnRH contains 10 peptides with a half-life of a few minutes. Exogenous GnRH agonists have an increased half-life of several hours due to increased lipophilicity. The continuous administration of GnRH agonists (daily or depot application) initially causes LH and FSH hypersecretion (flare), which is followed after a period of ~10 days by desensitization of the pituitary and profound suppression of LH and FSH. This results in the inhibition of ovarian steroidogenesis and follicular growth. The agonist may be used in a number of different protocols.

Short (flare)
- Agonist started on cycle day 1.
- 'Flare' of pituitary output of gonadotrophins.
- Exogenous gonadotrophins started on day 2.
- Agonist continued until day of hCG ('short' protocol) or for 3 days only ('ultrashort' protocol).

This protocol is sometimes used for women with reduced ovarian reserve. There is, however, no good evidence that this is better than other protocols, and it may be worse.

Microdose
- Theory is that reduced pituitary suppression will allow increased follicular response.
- Contraceptive pill pretreatment.
- Low dose of daily agonist started.

Long protocol
- Most established and widely used protocol.
- GnRH agonist suppresses pituitary production and release of gonadotrophins.
- Initially 'flare' of gonadotrophin release until suppression achieved.
- GnRH agonists can be given by depot injection, or daily s.c. or nasally, and commencing in either the mid-luteal or early follicular phase.
- Pituitary suppression generally achieved after 14–21 days. Confirmed by presence of withdrawal bleed, low serum oestradiol level (<150pmol/L) and/or ultrasound evidence of thin endometrium (<5mm). If not suppressed, then look for an ovarian cyst that will need to be aspirated (this may occur as the result of initial 'flare'). Alternatively high-dose progestagens can be administered which work by further suppressing pituitary gonadotrophin release. Despite prolonged administration of GnRH agonist ±cyst aspirations, some women fail to achieve pituitary suppression. Options include cancelling the cycle and restarting with antagonists.

Depot vs daily agonist treatment
- Depot agonist results in a more profound pituitary suppression. Consequently higher total doses of gonadotrophin are used and fewer oocytes retrieved.
- Women with nasal allergies or who sneeze soon after sniffing may prefer daily s.c. administration.

Mid-luteal vs early follicular agonist start
- Pregnancy rates are the same.
- Chance of starting agonist during a natural conception cycle with mid-luteal start. Has not been shown to be detrimental to the pregnancy.
- Higher rate of cyst formation with early follicular start.
- Cysts form in response to the initial 'flare' effect of the agonist. Inactive (no raised oestrogen level) cysts are not detrimental to outcome. If oestrogen level raised, then the cysts should be aspirated transvaginally under ultrasound guidance.

Antagonists
Unlike GnRH agonists, the antagonists do not induce an initial hyper-secretion of gonadotrophins, but instead cause an immediate and rapid, reversible suppression of gonadotrophin secretion. The principal mechanism of action of GnRH antagonists is competitive occupancy of the GnRH receptor. The administration of a third-generation antagonist (e.g. cetrorelix and ganirelix) will result in the suppression of LH (~70%) and FSH (~30%) serum levels after ~6h. The main benefits of antagonists over agonists are:

- No need for prolonged administration as with GnRH agonist since pituitary suppression achieved within hours of administration.
- Protocols are either flexible or fixed start and single or multiple dose. With flexible start, the antagonist is started when the leading follicle is 14mm diameter. With fixed start, the antagonist is started on day 7 of stimulation without using ultrasound monitoring (so regardless of follicular size). Whilst pregnancy rates are similar between the two approaches, the total gonadotrophin dose is higher with a fixed start.

Comparison of protocols (Cochrane reviews)

Depot GnRH agonist vs daily GnRH agonist

The use of a depot GnRH agonist compared with a daily agonist results in deeper pituitary suppression and an increased total dose of gonadotrophins, with a longer duration of stimulation but no difference in clinical pregnancy rates.

Antagonists vs agonists

The use of GnRH antagonists compared with agonists results in
- Lower rate of severe OHSS.
- Lower rate of coasting/cycle cancellation.
- Lower total dose and duration of gonadotrophin stimulation.
- Fewer oocytes collected.
- Possible lower rate of ongoing pregnancy/live births.

The reason for the lower pregnancy rate with antagonist cycles is not clear, but may be due to differences in endometrial quality.

Short agonist vs long agonist protocols

In unselected patients (i.e. not poor responders) the use of short (flare) protocols results in a significantly lower pregnancy rate.

Urinary-derived and recombinant gonadotrophins

Gonadotrophin preparations in use are either urinary derived or recombinant. The recombinant preparations are either pure FSH (follitropin-α or β) or pure LH. Urinary products contain different amounts of LH activity depending upon the particular preparation
- Urinary gonadotrophins are generally cheaper.
- There does not appear to be any difference between urinary or recombinant gonadotrophins in terms of live birth rate per cycle.
- There is a theoretical risk of prion transmission with the use of urinary drugs.

LH activity
- Some LH activity is required for optimal folliculogenesis (two-cell two-gonadotrophin model).
- Only 1% of follicular LH receptors need to be occupied for full LH effect.
- Therefore, the circulating levels of LH required are low.
- LH does not need to be added to stimulation protocols using recombinant FSH in women with an intact pituitary as pituitary suppression is not absolute.

- The degree of pituitary suppression is greater when depot GnRH agonist is used. Under these circumstances, some exogenous LH may be beneficial.
- Exogenous LH is needed for hypopituitary women (two-cell two-gonadotrophin model).

FSH dose selection

The main factors to consider with FSH dose selection are:
- Ovarian reserve. The lower the ovarian reserve, the higher the gonadotrophin dose.
- BMI. Overweight women require a higher dose.
- Previous ovarian response to stimulation including poor response and OHSS.
- Polycystic ovaries. The presence of ovaries of polycystic morphology, regardless of whether other aspects of the PCOS such as anovulation or hirsutism are present, is a risk factor for OHSS and so the FSH dose should be reduced. A starting dose of 150IU is prudent for the first cycle.

For women with normal ovarian reserve and without polycystic ovaries starting doses of 150–250IU result in similar numbers of oocytes retrieved and similar pregnancy rates.

Monitoring

- Monitoring of follicular response can be assessed with serum estradiol levels (which represents follicular granulosa cell activity) and the number and diameters of follicles measured with transvaginal ultrasound.
- The use of estradiol measurements in addition to scan monitoring does not improve the rates of pregnancy or reduce OHSS rates.

hCG is given when at least three follicles of ≥17–18mm diameter are present. The hCG mimics the mid-cycle LH surge. Recombinant LH is also available, though no advantages have been demonstrated.

Oocyte collection

In the early days of IVF, the oocyte collection was done laparoscopically and required general anaesthesia. Nowadays, oocyte aspiration is usually performed transvaginally under ultrasound guidance with i.v. sedation and analgesia, unless the ovary is not assessable by this route, or if gamete intrafallopian tube transfer (GIFT) is taking place. There still remains debate as to whether or not 'flushing' of the follicle in order to obtain more oocytes increases the pregnancy rate.

Embryo transfer and embryo freezing

This occurs usually on day 2 or 3 postoocyte insemination or ICSI. It may be delayed until blastocyst formation on day 5 in the attempt to select better morphological embryos and therefore improve the pregnancy rate per embryo transfer. The procedure involves passing a fine catheter through the cervix. This may be done under ultrasound control as this appears to increase the pregnancy rate. Replacement of embryos into a uterine cavity with an endometrium of <5mm thickness is unlikely to result in a pregnancy and is therefore not recommended.

Surplus embryos may be frozen and subsequently used in a frozen embryo replacement cycle (FERC). In general, the better the morphological quality of the embryo at freezing the better the survival rate from the freeze-thaw process. Pregnancy rates following FERCs tend to be 5–10% lower than the equivalent fresh embryo transfer cycle.

Luteal phase support

As a result of the downregulation of the hypothalamic–pituitary axis there will be insufficient endogenous LH to stimulate ovarian progesterone production following oocyte collection. Progesterone in the form of vaginal pessaries or i.m. injection will be required for the 2 weeks following oocyte collection and embryo transfer in order to ensure receptivity of the endometrium. The routine use of hCG (as an LH replacement) for luteal support is not recommended because of the increased likelihood of OHSS.

Intracytoplasmic sperm injection

This procedure was first carried out in 1993. Since that time, ICSI has been performed extensively. The recognized indications for treatment by ICSI include:

- Obstructive azoospermia.
- Non-obstructive azoospermia.

In addition, treatment by ICSI should be considered for couples in whom a previous IVF treatment cycle has resulted in failed or very poor fertilization. Before considering treatment by ICSI, couples should undergo appropriate investigations, both to establish a diagnosis and to enable informed discussion about the implications of treatment.

Where the indication for ICSI is a severe deficit of semen quality or non-obstructive azoospermia, the man's karyotype should be established. Where a specific genetic defect associated with male infertility is known or suspected (e.g. cystic fibrosis), couples should be offered appropriate genetic counselling and testing.

Testing for Y chromosome microdeletions should not be regarded as a routine investigation before ICSI. However, it is likely that a significant proportion of male infertility results from abnormalities of genes on the Y chromosome involved in the regulation of spermatogenesis, and couples should be informed of this.

Oocyte donation

The use of donor oocytes may be considered in managing fertility problems associated with the following conditions:
- premature ovarian failure.
- gonadal dysgenesis including Turner's syndrome.
- bilateral oophorectomy.
- ovarian failure following chemotherapy or radiotherapy.
- certain cases of IVF treatment failure where there is a severely diminished ovarian reserve.

Oocyte donation should also be considered in certain cases where there is a high risk of transmitting a genetic disorder to the offspring. Before donation is undertaken, oocyte donors should be screened for both infectious and genetic diseases. Oocyte donors should be offered information regarding the potential risks of ovarian stimulation and oocyte collection. Oocyte recipients and donors should be offered counselling regarding the physical and psychological implications of treatment for themselves and their genetic children, including any potential children resulting from donated oocytes.

'Egg-sharing' is a programme whereby women undergoing IVF offer to share half of the oocytes retrieved at collection with another women who requires egg donation. Both couples entering into this arrangement should be counselled about its particular implications.

Complications of IVF

The short-term risks of IVF include:
- OHSS.
- Trauma.
- Infection.
- Stress.

The most common problem is OHSS. Other less common complications are pelvic infection (0.4%), intraperitoneal bleeding (0.2%) and adnexal torsions (0.13%). Trauma accounts for ~0.1–0.2% and may involve problems such as puncture of an ovarian cyst, trauma to bowel, trauma to pelvic vessels and even trauma to the ureter.

Ovarian hyperstimulation syndrome (OHSS)

This is the best recognized complication of ovarian stimulation for IVF or ovulation induction. It remains incompletely understood, but the luteneizing trigger is undoubtedly an essential feature in the problem. If the luteinizing trigger is witheld, then the excessive ovarian response should regress without OHSS resulting. The worst cases tend to be associated with pregnancy since if there is no pregnancy the hCG stimulus soon regresses. Moderate OHSS occurs in ~3–4% of cycles, and risk of severe OHSS is ~0.1–0.2%. With the massive ovarian enlargement which occurs after luteinization in this syndrome, the clinical picture becomes complex. The problems include hypoproteinaemia, tension ascites, pleural effusion, haemoconcentration, oliguria and electolyte imbalance, a hypercoagulable state, liver dysfunction and, in some cases, deaths have occurred. Once the syndrome has developed, early admission is appropriate, but there are limited measures which can be employed. These include metabolic support with protein replacement to maintain the circulating volume, paracentesis to relieve the ascites and, in some very serious cases, termination of pregnancy.

Follow-up of children born as a result of Assisted reproduction

Follow-up of children born as a result of assisted reproduction

The course of pregnancies and the health of children born after assisted conception technologies are two of the most important outcome parameters of the quality of the techniques. There is ongoing discussion as to whether these parameters may show poorer results as compared with spontaneous conception. It was initially thought that this difference was predominantly the result of a higher incidence of multiple pregnancies in this group or the result of the increased maternal age. A recent study on subfecundity and neonatal outcome in the Danish national birth register also concluded that subfecundity in itself may be associated with an increased risk of neonatal death.

Shortly after its introduction in the mid 1990s, it was seen that children born following ICSI had a slightly increased incidence of abnormalities. On closer examination, it was seen that in the vast majority of these cases there was already an existing genetic or chromosomal predisposition in the paternal side.

It has been reported that genomic imprinting (an epigenetic phenomenon by which the expression of a gene is determined by its parental origin and only one allele of the imprinted gene is expressed) may be disrupted during IVF. It has been reported that Beckwith–Wiedemann syndrome (an imprinting disorder) has a 6-fold increase in incidence against a background incidence of ~1.3 per 100 000 newborns.

Whatever the factors are, it does appear that IVF pregnancies are at an increased risk of perinatal mortality and related perinatal outcomes (prematurity and low gestation weight). Whether these factors are related to aspects of the treatment or the underlying features that the couple bring to the pregnancy, or a mixture of both, is not yet clear.

Further reading and information

Human Fertilisation and Embryology Authority (HFEA): http://www.hfea.gov.uk/
National Institute for Health and Clinical Excellence (NICE) report into Fertility investigation and treatment: www.nice.org.uk/pdf/CG011niceguideline.pdf
Infertility network UK: http://www.infertilitynetworkuk.com/

Part II

Contraception and Family Planning

Fertility and fertility awareness

Introduction

We now shift to a consideration of 'the other side of the coin': fertility control rather than its enhancement. The authors consider it high time there was a medical text covering both: the clinical and research overlaps in both directions are rather obvious.

For example, sometimes women who have been warned (in terms that perhaps should have been more qualified) by a doctor about a possible threat to their future fertility (eg PCOS, or endometriosis) have misheard that to mean 'no need for any contraception': and have unwanted conceptions.

More often, clinically, other women after years of contraception then have difficulty in conceiving. Not unreasonably they may blame the contraceptive. Fortunately it is rare if it is ever that the methods *per se* are truly causative (beyond allowing the woman to get older before she 'tries'). Even the injectable DMPA is fully reversible, though in some it may considerably delay return of ovulation. Indeed it is *lack of* contraception leading to septic abortion that causes much (tubal) infertility, in some parts of the world—not to mention non-use of the condom causing pelvic inflammatory disease (PID) … .

From the research standpoint, it is a little disappointing that the fascinating new insights into reproductive biology that have been described above have, so far, largely failed to yield the expected dividends by 'being used in reverse': ie to create truly innovative, even hopefully 'ideal' (p. 264) contraceptives. But given the supreme urgency of the accelerating population/environment crisis, this can surely only be a matter of time. Watch this space!

Most women who seek contraception are healthy and young, and present fewer problems than the over-35s, teenagers and those with intercurrent disease. The combined oral contraceptive (COC) is too often seen as synonymous with contraception; there are, however, many new or improved reversible alternatives to the COC and the condom. The NICE Clinical Guideline 30 (www.nice.org.uk, 2005) drew attention to the many contraceptive (and sometimes non-contraceptive) advantages of the long-acting reversible contraceptives (LARCs): injectables, implants, the latest copper-banded IUDs and the levonorgestrel intra-uterine system (LNG-IUS).

Sex and Relationships Education (SRE)

Whether being taught or seeking advice on sex, relationships, contraception, pregnancy and parenthood, young people are entitled to:
- accessible
- confidential
- non-judgemental
- unbiased support and guidance that recognizes the diversity of their cultural and faith traditions.

Their own views should be listened to, respecting their own opinions and choices. Valid choices include what has been termed 'saving sex' (ie for another person, or another time) as well as having 'safer sex'.

The GMC has issued (2007) invaluable guidance focusing on children and young people from birth until their 18th birthday, concerning the standards of competence, care and conduct expected (of all doctors registered with the GMC). www.gmc-uk.org/guidance/ethical_guidance/children_guidance/index.asp

A significant proportion of early postpubertal menstrual cycles are not fertile. Hence adolescents who have unprotected sex shortly after puberty commonly 'get away with it': leading to a false sense of security later on, when their fertility is much higher. Typically also their pill-taking is very haphazard. Teenagers should therefore be offered one of the LARCs far more frequently than is currently the case in most settings, even if their first thought has been to ask for 'the Pill'. Injectables and implants are usually preferable to copper IUDs because they are more readily initiated (ie no vaginal procedure) and may provide some protection against pelvic infection—although IUDs are only relatively contraindicated. The LNG-IUS may also be appropriate.

Yet for many young women the most acceptable initial method of contraception currently remains either a modern, low-oestrogen COC or the new progestogen-only pill (POP).

With all these methods there should be appropriate condom advice along with preferably, on-the-spot supplies.

Patients under 16 years of age (age of consent)

Legally, following the Fraser Guidelines below (issued after the 1985 Gillick case), an attempt should first be made to involve a parent in the decision to prescribe a 'medical' method of contraception. Yet it can be good practice to prescribe, for example, the COC in the absence of such parental support.

• At all times the young person must be assured of confidentiality.
• Be alert for the possibility of abuse.

There is a useful mnemonic for the UK Memorandum of Guidance (DHSS HC (FP) 86) regarding under 16s (Fraser Guidelines):

Mnemonic: 'UnProtected SSexual InterCourse'

The health care practitioner:

U   Must ensure the young person **UNDERSTANDS** the potential risks and benefits of the treatment/advice given

P   Is legally obliged to discuss the value of **PARENTAL** support, yet the client must know that confidentiality is respected whether or not this is given

S   Should assess whether the client is likely to have **SEXUAL** intercourse without contraception

S   Should assess whether the young person's physical/mental health may **SUFFER** if not given contraceptive advice or supplies

I   Must consider if it is in the client's best **INTERESTS** to give contraception without parental consent

C   Must respect the duty of **CONFIDENTIALITY** that should be given to a person under 16, and which is as great as that owed to any other person.

If the above guidance is followed with utmost good faith, the prescription of a medical method of contraception will never be seen legally as aiding or abetting any crime.

Sexually transmitted infections

- The prevalence in the UK of all of these is rising.
- The most common conditions now are Chlamydia (>10% of sexually active teenagers have acquired *Chlamydia trachomatis*), non-specific urethritis and wart virus infections, but almost all sexually transmitted infections (STIs) are becoming more common.

In the UK, women at 'higher risk' of infection (particularly with *C. trachomatis*) are those:

- Aged under 25.
- A partner change in previous 12 weeks.
- More than one partner in past 12 months.

Sexual history should be seen as part of the initial consultation for *all* contraceptives, not just the intra-uterine ones:

- 'When did you last have sex?' followed at once by
- 'When did you last have sex with someone different?'

The sexually active of all ages should be advised about minimizing their risk of STIs, including the human immunodeficiency virus (HIV). *It is essential to promote the condom as an addition to the selected contraceptive, whenever infection risk exists.*

Contact tracing

Where an STI has been identified, contact screening is best done through a Genitourinary Medicine (GUM) clinic. If a patient refuses, then give the patient a letter to give to contacts stating the disease that they have been in contact with and suggesting that they attend a GUM clinic.

Features of the ideal contraceptive

Consideration of the factors affecting successful use of contraception by young people lends support to the need for as many as possible of the 10 features listed below

The ideal contraceptive

- 100% effective (with the default state as contraception).
- 100% convenient (forgettable, non-coitally related).
- 100% safe, free of adverse side-effects (neither risk nor nuisance).
- 100% reversible, ideally by self.
- 100% maintenance free, meaning needing absolutely no medical or provider intervention (with potential pain or discomfort): whether initially, or during usage, or to achieve reversal.
- 100% protective against STIs.
- Having other non-contraceptive benefits, especially to the dis-'eases' of the menstrual cycle.
- Cheap, easy to distribute.
- Acceptable to every culture, religion and political view.
- Used by or at least clearly visible to the woman, who most needs to know it has worked!

It is difficult to decide the best priority order for these, though the first six bullets are clearly paramount.

To date, the nearest approach to the ideal that we have is arguably the LNG-IUS (see 📖 **p. 402, where its few shortcomings are discussed).**

Relative effectiveness of the available methods

Failure rates of contraceptive methods are usually expressed as failures per 100 woman-years. A figure of 10 per 100 woman-years for a 'perfect user' (see below) means:

- in a population of 100 users 10 women might be expected to conceive in the first year of use
- or one woman would have an 'evens' chance of having an unplanned pregnancy after 10yrs of its use.

In Table 19.1 'Perfect use' means the method is used both consistently and correctly, whereas 'Typical use' means what it says—and note the huge difference in percentage conceiving after 1yr between the two types of use for the combined pill (0.3 vs 8).

Fig. 19.1 shows current usage of the present 'mix' of methods in the UK.

Table 19.1 Percentage of women experiencing an unintended pregnancy during the first year of use (Data from United States of America)

Method	Typical use	Perfect use
No method	85	85
Spermicides	29	18
Withdrawal	27	4
Periodic abstinence	25	
Calendar		9
Ovulation method		3
Sympto-thermal[1]		2
Postovulation		1
Cap+spermicide		
Parous women	32	26
Nulliparous women	16	9
Sponge		
Parous women	32	20
Nulliparous women	16	9
Diaphragm	16	6
Condom		
Female	21	5
Male	15	2
Combined pill and minipill	8	0.3
Combined hormonal patch	8	0.3
Combined hormonal ring	8	0.3
DMPA	3	0.3
Combined injectable	3	0.05
IUD		
ParaGard® (banded copper T)	0.8	0.6
Mirena® (LNG-IUS)	0.1	0.1
LNG implants	0.05	0.05
Female sterilization	0.5	0.5
Male sterilization	0.15	0.1

Emergency contraceptive pills: treatment initiated within 72 h after unprotected intercourse reduces the risk of pregnancy by at least 75%.
Lactational amenorrhoea method: LAM is a highly effective, *temporary method* of contraception

Source: Trussell J. Contraceptive efficacy. In: Hatcher RA, Trussell J, Stewart F, Nelson A, Cates W, Guest F, Kowal D. *Contraceptive Technology: Eighteenth Revised Edition*. New York NY: Ardent Media, 2004.

Note: This table in WHOMEC, 3rd Edition, 2004, has been adapted from the source document by changing the title, changing the trade names of methods to generic names and by modifying footnotes.

[1] This refers to the cervical mucus method supplemented by calendar calculation in the preovulatory and basal body temperature charting in the postovulatory phases. See 📖 p. 272.

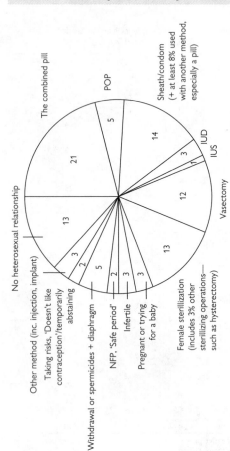

Fig. 19.1 Current contraceptive usage in the UK. Derived from the Omnibus Survey of the Office for National Statistics from a stratified random sample of individuals surveyed up to March 2005. (Adjusted by the author so far as feasible for respondents giving >1 answer.) Note: emergency contraception was also mentioned by 1%, but presumably coming into another category for the rest of their current sex lives (e.g. abstaining, condoms, etc.)

Source: National Statistics website: www.statistics.gov.uk

Eligibility criteria for contraceptives

The World Health Organization (WHO) system for classifying contraindications

The World Health Organization (WHO) system for classifying contraindications is described in the documents issued by WHO, *Medical Eligibility Criteria for Contraceptive Use* (WHOMEC)(3rd edn, 2004, ISBN: 92 4 156266 8) and *Selected Practice Recommendations for Contraceptive Use* (WHOSPR)(ISBN: 92 4 154566 6): www.who.int/reproductive-health.

In 2006 the Faculty of Family Planning and Reproductive Healthcare (FFPRHC) issued UKMEC, a UK-adapted version of WHOMEC developed by its Clinical Effectiveness Unit. This version, downloadable from http://www.ffprhc.org.uk, is the one generally used here.

On several issues where UKMEC has not yet given its verdict, or where other authorities differ from WHO, this book attempts to give best interim guidance according to this author's judgement of the evidence—but using the same four categories of contraindication (see the box on 📖 p. 271).

WHO classification of contraindications (amplified by the author)

WHO 1. A condition for which there is no restriction for the use of the contraceptive method

'A' is for Always Usable

WHO 2. A condition where the advantages of the method generally outweigh the theoretical or proven risks

'B' is for Broadly Usable

****

WHO 3. A condition where the theoretical or proven risks usually outweigh the advantages, so an alternative method is usually preferred. Yet, respecting the patient/client's autonomy, if she accepts the risks and rejects or should not use relevant alternatives, given the risks of pregnancy the method can be used with caution/sometimes with additional monitoring

'C' is for 'Caution/Counselling', if used at all

WHO 4. A condition which represents an unacceptable health risk

'D' is for 'DO NOT USE', at all

Clinical judgement is required, always in consultation with the contraceptive user, especially: (1) in all WHO 3 conditions; or (2) if more than one condition applies. As a working rule, two WHO 2 conditions move the situation to WHO 3; and if any WHO 3 condition applies, the addition of either a 2 or a 3 condition normally means WHO 4, i.e. 'Do not use'.

Fertility awareness and methods for the natural regulation of fertility

These are capable of being much more reliable than the old calendar rhythm (see the excellent website www.fertilityuk.org and associated review by Pyper and Knight[1]) if there is correct and consistent use. However, they still remain 'very unforgiving of imperfect use'.

Short notes on the background physiology

- An average fertile man's ejaculate contains ~300–400 million sperm.
- The acidic vaginal environment can kill sperm in a matter of hours; however, in oestrogen-primed cervical mucus and upper genital tract fluid, *average* sperm survival is ~3 days.
- In rare individuals or rare cycles in which favourable mucus appears early, *fertilization can be as long as* **7 days** *after ejaculation.*
- The average fertilizable lifespan of the egg(s) after ovulation is ~17h, with a range up to a maximum of 24h.
- Adding the lifetime of the sperm to that of the egg gives a 'fertile window' of 7–8 days, whose length is rather constant; but its time of onset shows intra- as well as inter-individual variation.
- Maximum reliability will require many days of abstinence, especially early in the cycle. For maximum efficacy with any of the methods, unprotected intercourse should preferably, following good evidence of ovulation, be confined to the days after the ovum is no longer fertilizable.

The markers of ovulation

- A rise in basal temperature which has been sustained for 72h at least 0.2°C above the preceding 6 days' values.
- Observations of the mucus as detected at the vulva. This becomes increasingly fluid, glossy, transparent, slippery and stretchy, like raw egg white, under the influence of follicular oestrogen. The peak mucus day can be recognized retrospectively as the last day with such features before the abrupt change to a thick and tacky type (under the influence of progesterone).

The postovulatory infertile phase is defined as beginning on the evening of the 4th day after the peak mucus day, provided this is also after the third of the higher morning temperature readings.

Relying on *both* the above signals for the onset of the postovulatory infertile phase and using that alone for unprotected intercourse can give very acceptable failure rates of 1–3 per 100 woman-years.

[1] Pyper CM, Knight J. Fertility awareness methods of family planning: the physiological background, methodology and effectiveness of fertility awareness methods. *J Fam Plann Reprod Health Care* 2001; **27**: 103–110.

The preovulatory infertile phase is much more difficult to identify with accuracy. The indicators are:
- the first sign of any mucus at all, detected by either sensation or appearance;
- calendar calculation of the shortest cycle minus 20 (or better, 21) to give the last 'infertile' day: where at least six cycle lengths are known. This can be enhanced by the Doering rule in which 7 days are subtracted from the earliest cycle day of documented temperature shift. Whichever of these two indicators comes first indicates the requirement to abstain.

Relying on both phases is only to be recommended to those who can accept a pregnancy, since calculations and mucus observations do NOT reliably predict ovulation far enough ahead to eliminate (over many months or years) the capricious survival of that last-surviving sperm which could cause conception.

The postpartum period and in the climacteric years

Temperature and mucus estimations are unreliable and/or give numerous 'false alarms', since some cycles are anovulatory yet still there is sufficient oestrogen to produce slippery mucus.

Postcontraceptive hormone use

The indicators are also unreliable here and it is advised that this 'symptom-thermal' approach—or the use of Persona® (below)—is deferred, even following hormonal emergency contraception, until there have been at least two subsequent bleeds, along with initial reliance on the postovulation phase.

Advantages of methods based on fertility awareness
- They are completely free from any known physical side-effects for the user.
- They are acceptable to many with certain religious and cultural views, not only Roman Catholics.
- The methods are under the couple's personal control (abstinence is always available!).
- The methods readily lend themselves, if the couple's scruples permit, to the additional use of an artificial method such as a barrier at the potentially fertile times, including during the less safe first 'infertile' phase.
- Once established as efficient users, after proper teaching, no further expensive follow-up of the couple is necessary.
- Understanding of the methods can also help couples who then wish to conceive.

Problems and disadvantages
- In practice, *typical use* gives very high failure rates (25 per 100 woman-years according to Trussell, Table 19.1). This is almost entirely due to rule breaking.
- Conflicts and frustrations are reported, though interestingly enough, the majority of *established* users believe the method to be helpful to their marriage/relationship rather than stressing it.

- A potential hazard is fetal abnormalities due to conceptions tending to result from fertilization involving ageing gametes. The consensus after a number of studies is that this risk, if real, is negligible.

Useful instruction leaflets, further advice and details of Natural Family Planning (NFP) teachers who are available in different localities—mostly outside the NHS—can be obtained from:

Fertility UK
Bury Knowle Health Centre
207 London Road
Headington
Oxford OX3 9JA
E-mail: admin@fertility uk.org
   www.fertilityuk.org

The fpa
51 Featherstone Street
London EC1Y 8QU
Helpline Tel: 0845 310 1334
www.fpa.org.uk

'PERSONA®—the Unipath personal contraceptive system
This innovative product, first marketed in 1996, consists of a number of disposable test sticks and a hand-held, computerized monitor. As instructed by the device, the test sticks are dipped in the user's early morning urine samples and transferred to a slot in the device where the levels of both oestrone 3-glucuronide (E-3-G) and LH are measured by a patented immunochromatographic assay, utilizing an optical monitor.
- When a significant increase in the E-3-G level is detected, the fertility status is changed to 'unsafe', i.e. a *red* light replaces the *green* one on the monitor.
- After subsequent detection of the first significant rise of LH, the end of the fertile period is not signalled by a *green* light until a further 4 days have elapsed.

The system also stores and utilizes data on the individual's previous six menstrual cycles.

Efficacy information suggests a failure rate in consistent users no better than 6 per 100 woman-years, i.e. not as good as the best rates reported by perfect users of the symptom-thermal or multiple index methods.

Advantages
- Persona® is much simpler and quicker to use; no charting, etc. required
- Less abstinence: a 'fertile' period lasting ≤8 days was signalled to 80% of users, and this is a definite improvement on the 10–12 days' abstinence usually demanded by the multiple index methods.

For greater efficacy, it is worth suggesting to some couples that they consider using condoms very carefully in the first 'green' phase, abstinence in the 'red' phase and unprotected intercourse only in the second 'green' phase. This approach should reduce the failure rate to the best reported above, but has not been formally tested.

The lactational amenorrhoea method (LAM)

Ovulation is delayed among women who fully or nearly fully breastfeed their babies. It usually takes between 1 and 3 months for a woman to begin to ovulate and for her cycle to return to normal after stopping breastfeeding. LAM is an algorithm, as shown in Fig. 19.2, allowing a woman to determine whether she is comfortable to rely on her pattern of infant feeding and menstruation to predict anovulation or should add an additional method of contraception.

Additional methods for post partum use

- The COC should be avoided in lactation as it may inhibit this and also alter the quality of the milk. Otherwise the COC is a suitable choice post partum.
- The POP is preferable, in the UK usually started like the COC on day 21, though WHOSPR recommends later (6 weeks) for ALL hormonal methods. This does not interfere significantly with lactation and, although traces may enter the milk, the quantity has been calculated (see POP section below) as equivalent to a baby getting just one pill over 2 years.
- Spermicides or contraceptive sponges, though not generally effective enough for recommendation to young people, are strong enough as adjunctive methods while the LAM rules are valid.
- Condoms (including the female condom) are useful for first intercourse postpartum and until other methods are established. Caps and diaphragms may be refitted at 5–6 weeks, and this is always necessary after a full-term pregnancy, even after Caesarean section.
- The injectable, DMPA (depot medroxyprogesterone acetate), aside from slightly higher milk levels (which seem to be harmless to the infant), may be a preferable progestogen-only method for women who might be short-term breastfeeders and unreliable POP takers, but want high efficacy right through weaning and thereafter. It does no detect-able harm to the quality and may even improve the quantity of the breast milk.
- Implanon® is another option despite the caution of the SPC. WHOSPR recommends method commencement at 6 weeks in breastfeeders, as for DMPA (and POPs).
- The IUD or IUS are easily inserted at 4–6 weeks postpartum or 6–8 weeks after a Caesarean section, but the uterus is still soft and great care is necessary. Earlier insertion is more likely to lead to expulsion.
- Sterilization procedures performed in the post partum period carry extra operative, failure rate, and emotional risks (including greater risk of regret). Surgery for either partner is usually, and preferably, delayed for a few months.

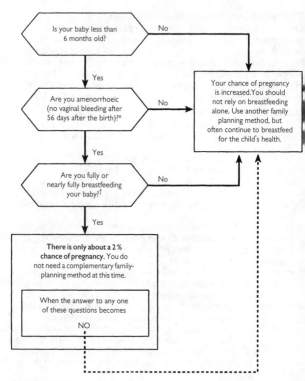

Fig. 19.2 Algorithm for the lactational amenorrhoea method (LAM). *Spotting that occurs during the first 56 days is not considered to be menstruation. 'Nearly' full breastfeeding means that the baby obtains 100% of its nutrition from the mother alone, and certainly no solid food.

Reproduced from *The Pill* part of the Facts series. 6th edition. By permission of Oxford University Press.

Male contraception

Coitus interruptus

The earliest form of reversible birth control (mentioned in Genesis and positively in Islamic texts); it is well described by its most common euphemism, 'withdrawal' (before ejaculation, ensuring that all sperm are deposited outside the vagina).

Effectiveness of coitus interruptus

In 1949 the UK Royal Commission on Population reported the pregnancy rate as 8 per 100 woman-years of exposure. Trussell gives a 4% failure rate in the first year of 'perfect use' (see Table 19.1).

Sperm are found at low density in some men in the pre-ejaculate. A more probable cause of failure is the partial ejaculation of a larger quantity of semen, either occurring a short while before the final male orgasm; or withdrawal during the latter rather than before it starts.

It can therefore be useful to advise couples who want to continue using the method that they might use a spermicide as well (never instead).

Advantages
- Free, requires no prescription.
- Always available.
- No side-effects.

Disadvantages
- Intercourse is incomplete, and either or both partners may find the method decidedly unsatisfying.

Conclusion

Coitus interruptus is almost never proposed to a couple. If they volunteer that this is already their usual method, other options should always be discussed. If all alternatives are unacceptable, then the additional use of spermicide (e.g. as a pessary or sponge) should be suggested.

Male condoms

Condoms are the only proven barrier to transmission of HIV. Condom are second in usage to the COC under the age of 30 and to sterilizatic above that age.

Effectiveness

- 'Perfect use': failure rate of 2%, and typical use leads to 15% conceivin in the first year.

The main reason for failure is either intermittent non-use or incorre use: mainly through the escape of a small amount of semen either befo or after the condom is in place for the main ejaculation, rather tha rupture.

Advantages and indications

Advantages aside from acceptable, *potentially* good, efficacy include:
- Useful protection against all STIs including HIV and human papilloma virus (HPV).
- Easy to obtain, even at odd hours.
- User (man) takes responsibility; no inconvenient need to see a health service provider.
- No medical risks and no supervision required.
- Visual proof of having 'worked'.
- Helps delay some with premature ejaculation.
- Good for infrequent intercourse.
- For women who dislike the smell or messiness of semen, the condom solves their problem.

Problems and disadvantages

- To many, condoms seem intrusive; alteration of sensations in the penetrative phase of sex are reported by the male, sometimes by both partners.
- Poor efficacy in typical use, largely from lack of care or consistency— often related to first bullet above. Hence often best *combined* with a 'medical' and more effective method.
- Needs to be available … more forward planning needed than some can manage!
- Can slip off or rupture in use.
- Some older men, or younger but with sexual anxiety, find that condom use may result in loss of erection. This sometimes provides enough grounds to prescribe sildenafil.
- The rubber smell can be off-putting and true allergy can occur (rarely both problems that can be completely solved by switching to plastic condoms (e.g. Avanti® or Ez-On®). The latter also avoid the next risk in this list.
- Rubber (not plastic) condoms may be seriously weakened by oil-base chemicals. All users need warning of this risk. Water-based and silicor lubricants are OK.

Lubricants with the spermicide nonoxinol 9 should be avoided with any condom, since it is now evidence-based that it can increase HIV transmission (see below)—moreover it provides no detectable increase in condom efficacy.

The Ez-On® condom and its variants

Available in California and The Netherlands, this is plastic, loose-fitting and well-lubricated: the 'looks funny, feels good' condom. By better simulating the normal vagina, it is designed to overcome the undeniable interference with penile sensation that condoms may cause, during the penetrative phase of intercourse.

The male Pill

The male pill is still very much a work in progress and has yet to be marketed. The main problems are:
- Male contraception is biologically more difficult to achieve than female contraception. There is no single regular event like ovulation which can be stopped.
- A 'male pill' must not affect libido, must give extremely good protection against pregnancy and be as free as possible from side-effects.
- There is a special risk here too that interference with the production of the sperm might be incomplete. So if one sperm were to be *damaged* by whatever the treatment might be, yet managed to fertilize an egg, this might result in a birth defect.
- Spermatogenesis takes ~70 days. Thus any male pill operating on this manufacturing process will take at least 2 months to become effective. It also means that there must be a long recovery period after stopping the method.

Research has focused either on:
- stopping the production of sperm or
- inactivating or blocking them once produced.

The former approach is the closest to producing a viable, marketed method, by combining a progestogen by injection or implant with an androgen, a long-acting analogue of testosterone. This blocks both FSH and LH, the latter therefore switching off production of testosterone: but the androgen content is titrated to a level to preserve libido and drive without the latter turning into aggression.

Vasectomy

There is more about male as well as female sterilization in Chapter 28.

Bilateral vasectomy is a safe and effective method of male sterilization. In the UK, ~23% of couples of reproductive age choose vasectomy as their method of contraception. Because the sperm itself makes up a very small proportion of an ejaculation, vasectomy does not significantly affect the volume, appearance, texture or flavour of the ejaculate. Two negative semen analyses (2–4 weeks apart and >12 weeks since the procedure) are the norm after the surgical procedure to ensure effectiveness.

In counselling, several steps are necessary before valid consent can be obtained. See Chapter 28. The process should at least include:
- An assessment of the patient's contraceptive needs, and discussion of alternative methods.
- A general discussion of the surgical technique, tailored to the individual.
- A frank and honest discussion of the risks and specific complications associated with vasectomy.
- As with any medical intervention, only patients of sound mind and capable of understanding these issues are able to give valid consent.

Early failure rates of vasectomy are generally <1%, but the effectiveness of the operation and rates of complications vary with the level of experience of the surgeon performing the operation and the surgical technique used. Although late failure (caused by recanalization of the vasa deferentia) is very rare, it has been documented.

Failure rates (first year)	
Perfect use	<0.1%
Typical use	0.15%
Usage	
Duration effect	Permanent
Reversibility	Often, but not always
User reminders	Additional methods required until two negative semen samples
Clinic review	None

Vaginal methods

Female condoms

Femidom® is the UK-marketed variety of female condom comprising a polyurethane sac with an outer rim at the introitus and a loose inner ring, whose retaining action is similar to that of the rim of the diaphragm. It thus forms a well-lubricated (with silicone) secondary vagina.

- Effectiveness: failure rate 5% among 'perfect' users after one year.
- Duration of use: used near or at the time of intercourse, whereas the diaphragm or cap must be left in place for at least 6h after intercourse. Appropriate for both short-term and long-term use. Reuse of the female condom is not recommended. Women can use barrier contraceptives throughout their reproductive years.
- Parity limitations: no restrictions on use for nulliparous or parous women, although parous women may experience higher rates of pregnancy with the diaphragm and cap.

Advantages

- Useful protection against all STIs including HIV and HPV.
- Available over the counter, along with a well-illustrated leaflet.
- Completely resistant to damage by any chemicals with which it might come into contact.
- Usable where either party is allergic to rubber.
- The penetrative phase of intercourse can feel more normal to a man than when a male condom is used.
- Uniquely among condoms, it can be put in place before the man has an erection.

Disadvantages

Couples should be forewarned of:

- The definite possibility that the penis may become wrongly positioned between the Femidom® sac and the vaginal wall.
- Its obviousness particularly during foreplay.

Caps and diaphragms

These create a vaginal barrier to sperm either in the upper vagina (diaphragms) or at the cervix itself (caps of varying design, though since mid-2007 Fem Cap® is the only one on the UK market).

- Effectiveness: failure rate 5 per 100 'perfect' users, rising to 16 per 100 typical users after one year.

Advantages

- Once initiated, many couples express surprise at the simplicity of these vaginal barriers. They are best reserved for couples in a stable relationship where sexual activity takes on a relatively regular pattern, and conception would not be seen as a disaster.
- All may be inserted well ahead of coitus, and so used without spoiling spontaneity.
- There is very little reduction in sexual sensitivity, as the clitoris and introitus are not affected and cervical pressure is still possible.

Disadvantages

- Rather moderate efficacy, plus lack of complete protection against the viral STIs such as HIV.
- Concerns about spermicide safety (see below).
- Perceptions that they are a hassle to learn to use.

Spermicide is recommended for use as well, because no mechanical barrier is complete. Possible toxic effects of nonoxinol—which is unfortunately the only spermicidal agent marketed in UK—to the vaginal wall have now become a real concern (see below).

Fitting and follow-up

- One-to-one training is crucial, both in the process of fitting the diaphragm and cervical caps, and in teaching a woman how to use it correctly, backed up by an appropriate leaflet.
- The fitting of diaphragms should be checked initially after 1–2 weeks of trial and re-checked routinely postpartum, or whenever there is more than 3kg gain or loss in weight.
- If either partner returns complaining that they can feel a diaphragm during coitus, the fitting must be urgently checked. It could be too large or too small; or the retro-pubic ledge may be insufficient to prevent the front slipping down the anterior vagina; or, most seriously with respect to efficacy, the item may be being regularly placed in the anterior fornix.

Recurrent cystitis may be linked to pressure from a diaphragm's anterior rim, and hence often improves with a *vault* or *cervical cap* (now referring only to FemCap®), which does not apply pressure on the anterior vagina.

Spermicide (nonoxinol)

Although invaluable as an adjunct to caps and diaphragms and for some couples using coitus interruptus long term, spermicide used alone—whether as creams, jellies, pessaries or foams—is simply not acceptably reliable. However, good effectiveness has been reported in women whose fertility is already reduced (see box).

Contraceptive sponges are expected back on the UK market in 2008 as the Today™ sponge, and they share the advantage with spermicides of being sexually very convenient and unobtrusive in use, but once again lack sufficient efficacy (Table 21.1) for acceptability by most young, fertile women. Yet all these methods can be good for defined populations (see box)

The Today™ sponge when available or other spermicidal products may be good choices in the following cases:
- For women >50yrs of age if still experiencing bleeds after stopping the COC (see 🕮 p. 433) and for 1yr after the menopause (i.e. the duration for which contraception is still advised) whether or not they use HRT.
- For women aged >45 if they have oligo-amenorrhoea.
- During lactation, as an alternative to the POP.
- During continuing 2° amenorrhoea, unless a COC is being used anyway to treat hypo-oestrogenism.
- As an adjunct to other contraception, e.g. spermicides may be useful as a supplement in couples who choose to continue using coitus interruptus/withdrawal as their main method.
- For those who are nearly but not quite ready for a first or subsequent child.

Table 21.1 Percentage of women experiencing an unintended pregnancy during the first year of use (Data from United States of America)

Method	Typical use	Perfect use
No method	85	85
Spermicides	29	18
Withdrawal	27	4
Periodic abstinence	25	
Calendar		9
Ovulation method		3
Sympto-thermal[1]		2
Postovulation		1
Cap+spermicide		
Parous women	32	26
Nulliparous women	16	9
Sponge		
Parous women	32	20
Nulliparous women	16	9
Diaphragm	16	6
Condom		
Female	21	5
Male	15	2
Combined pill and minipill	8	0.3
Combined hormonal patch	8	0.3
Combined hormonal ring	8	0.3
DMPA	3	0.3
Combined injectable	3	0.05
IUD		
ParaGard® (banded copper T)	0.8	0.6
Mirena® (LNG-IUS)	0.1	0.1
LNG implants	0.05	0.05
Female sterilization	0.5	0.5
Male sterilization	0.15	0.1

Emergency contraceptive pills: treatment initiated within 72h after unprotected intercourse reduces the risk of pregnancy by at least 75%.
Lactational amenorrhoea method: LAM is a highly effective, *temporary method* of contraception

Source: Trussell J. Contraceptive efficacy. In: Hatcher RA, Trussell J, Stewart F, Nelson A, Cates W, Guest F, Kowal D. *Contraceptive Technology: Eighteenth Revised Edition*. New York NY: Ardent Media, 2004.

Note: This table in WHOMEC, 3rd Edition, 2004, has been adapted from the source document by changing the title, changing the trade names of methods to generic names and by modifying footnotes.

[1] This refers to the cervical mucus method supplemented by calendar calculation in the preovulatory and basal body temperature charting in the postovulatory phases. See 📖 p. 272.

Disadvantages

- The currently available spermicide, nonoxinol, is certainly absorbed from the vagina, but there is no proof of systemic harm, congenital malformations or spontaneous abortions as a result
- Occasionally, sensitivity to spermicide arises.
- More seriously, when used by Nairobi sex workers four times a day for 14 days, nonoxinol released from pessaries caused erythema and colposcopic evidence of minor damage to the vaginal skin. Subsequent clinical trials have confirmed an increased risk of HIV transmission with use of spermicidal products using nonoxinol[1]. High risk of HIV infection is therefore WHO 4 (see 📖 p. 271) for this substance whether used alone or with a vaginal barrier.

However, the vagina is believed to be able to recover between applications when nonoxinol is used in the manner, and at the kind of average coital frequency, of appropriately counselled diaphragm or cap users. So it remains good practice to continue to recommend nonoxinol-9 for normal contraceptive use, whether alone or with diaphragms or cervical caps; but not with condoms (📖 p. 281).

1 Wilkinson D, Tholandi M, Ramjee G, Rutherford GW. Nonoxynol-9 spermicide for prevention of vaginally acquired HIV and other sexually transmitted infections: systematic review and meta-analysis of randomised controlled trials including more than 5000 women. *Lancet Infect Dis* 2002; 2: 613–617.

The combined oral contraceptive (COC)

Mechanism of action

- Primarily prevents ovulation.
- Secondary contraceptive effects on the cervical mucus and to impede implantation.

This makes the method highly effective in 'perfect' use (Table 22.1); but it removes the normal menstrual cyle and replaces it with a cycle which is user-produced and based only on the end-organ, i.e. the endometrium. So the withdrawal bleeding has minimal medical significance, can be deliberately postponed or made infrequent (e.g. tricycling; the taking of three consecutive packets thereby reducing withdrawal bleed frequency) and, if it fails to occur, once pregnancy is excluded, poses no problem. The pill-free time is the contraception-deficient time, which has great relevance to advice for the maintenance of the COC's efficacy (see below).

Table 22.1 Percentage of women experiencing an unintended pregnancy during the first year of use (Data from United States of America)

Method	Typical use	Perfect use
No method	85	85
Spermicides	29	18
Withdrawal	27	4
Periodic abstinence	25	
Calendar		9
Ovulation method		3
Sympto-thermal[1]		2
Postovulation		1
Cap+spermicide		
Parous women	32	26
Nulliparous women	16	9
Sponge		
Parous women	32	20
Nulliparous women	16	9
Diaphragm	16	6
Condom		
Female	21	5
Male	15	2
Combined pill and minipill	8	0.3
Combined hormonal patch	8	0.3
Combined hormonal ring	8	0.3
DMPA	3	0.3
Combined injectable	3	0.05
IUD		
ParaGard® (banded copper T)	0.8	0.6
Mirena® (LNG-IUS)	0.1	0.1
LNG implants	0.05	0.05
Female sterilization	0.5	0.5
Male sterilization	0.15	0.1

Emergency contraceptive pills: treatment initiated within 72h after unprotected intercourse reduces the risk of pregnancy by at least 75%.
Lactational amenorrhoea method: LAM is a highly effective, *temporary method of contraception*

Source: Trussell J. Contraceptive efficacy. In: Hatcher RA, Trussell J, Stewart F, Nelson A, Cates W, Guest F, Kowal D. *Contraceptive Technology: Eighteenth Revised Edition.* New York NY: Ardent Media, 2004.

Note: This table in WHOMEC, 3rd Edition, 2004, has been adapted from the source document by changing the title, changing the trade names of methods to generic names and by modifying footnotes.

[1] This refers to the cervical mucus method supplemented by calendar calculation in the preovulatory and basal body temperature charting in the postovulatory phases. See p. 272.

Benefits versus risks

Contraceptive benefits of COCs
- Effectiveness.
- Convenience, not intercourse related, 'forgettability'.
- Reversibility.

Non-contraceptive benefits of COCs—*which at times may provide the principal indication for use of the method (e.g. in the treatment of dysmenorrhoea in a not yet sexually active teenager).*
- Reduction of most menstrual cycle disorders: less heavy bleeding, therefore less anaemia, and less dysmenorrhoea; regular bleeding, the timing of which can be controlled (no COC taker need have 'periods' at weekends; upon request, she may tricycle and so bleed only a few times a year): fewer symptoms of premenstrual tension overall; no ovulation pain.
- Reduced risk of cancers of ovary and endometrium (see text), and now very probably also colorectal cancer.
- Fewer functional ovarian cysts because abnormal ovulation is prevented.
- Fewer extra-uterine pregnancies because normal ovulation is inhibited.
- Reduction in pelvic inflammatory disease (PID).
- Reduction in benign breast disease.
- Fewer symptomatic fibroids.
- Probable reduction in thyroid disease, whether over- or underactive.
- Probable reduction in risk of rheumatoid arthritis.
- Fewer sebaceous disorders (with oestrogen-dominant COCs).
- Possibly fewer duodenal ulcers (not well established).
- Reduction in *Trichomonas vaginalis* infections.
- Possible lower incidence of toxic shock syndrome.
- Continuous use beneficial in long-term suppression of endometriosis
- No toxicity in overdose.
- Some obvious beneficial social effects, to balance suggested negatives.

Risks of COCs
- Tumours: breast, cervical, liver.
- Venous thromboembolism (VTE).
- Arterial diseases: acute myocardial infarction (AMI), haemorrhagic stroke (HS) and ischaemic stroke (IS).

Tumour risk and COCs

Breast cancer

COC users can be reassured that:

- An odds ratio of 1.24 signifies an increase of 24% only while women are taking the COC, diminishing to zero after discontinuation, over the next few years.
- Beyond 10yrs after stopping, there is no detectable increase in breast cancer risk for former COC users.
- The cancers diagnosed in women who use or have ever used COCs are clinically less advanced than in those who have never used COCs, and are less likely to have spread beyond the breast.
- These risks are not associated with duration of use, the dose or type of hormone in the COC, and there is no synergism with other risk factors for breast cancer (e.g. family history). See Table 22.2.
- If 1000 women use the pill till age 35, by age 45 this model shows there will be, in all, 11 cases of breast cancer. Importantly, however, only one of these cases is extra (pill-related); the others would have arisen in a control group of never-users.

Table 22.2 The increased risk of developing breast cancer while taking the pill and in the 10yrs after stopping

User status	Increased risk
Current user	24%
1–4yrs after stopping	16%
5–9yrs after stopping	7%
10yrs + an ex-user	No significant excess

Reprinted with permission from Elsevier (*The Lancet*, 1996, Vol 360, 📖 pp. 1803–10).

Clinical implications

Women with benign breast disease (BBD) or *with the family history of a young first-degree relative with breast cancer under age 40.*

- Have a larger background risk than the generality of women, but only the same as women slightly older than their current age who are free of the risk factor. WHOMEC classifies both these conditions as WHO 1 for the COC (no restriction to use).
- If the woman with BBD had a breast biopsy, the histology should be obtained: if epithelial atypia (premalignant) was found, the situation for the COC changes to WHO 4.
- If a woman develops carcinoma of the breast, COCs should be discontinued, and women with a history of this cancer should normally avoid COCs (WHO 4).

Cervical cancer

COC acts as a cofactor for the human papilloma virus (HPV) types 16 and 18, the principal carcinogen in cervical cancer, speeding transition through the stages of cervical intraepithelial neoplasia (CIN). In this respect it is similar to, but certainly weaker than, cigarette smoking.

Clinical implications

Prescribers must ensure that COC users are adequately screened following agreed guidelines.

It is acceptable practice (WHO 2) to continue COC use during the careful monitoring of any abnormality, or after definitive treatment of CIN.

Liver tumours

Increased relative risk of **benign adenoma** or **hamartoma**. However, the background incidence is so small (1–3 per 1 million women per year) that the COC-attributable risk is minimal.

Three case–control studies also support the view that the rare **primary hepatocellular carcinoma** is minimally less rare in COC users than it is in controls.

Clinical implications: a past history of either tumour is WHO 4 for the COC but WHO 3 for other forms of hormonal contraception (WHOMEC).

Choriocarcinoma or, more generally, all gestational trophoblastic disease

Some evidence suggesting very slight increase in incidence, but not conclusive evidence. In the UK, although WHOMEC classifies this as WHO 1, when any form of trophoblastic disease has been diagnosed it is still recommended, by UKMEC and the UK regional centres that monitor all cases, that so long as hCG levels are raised the COC should be avoided (WHO 4). There is a theoretical risk of inducing metastatic disease or drug-resistant disease. *But thereafter the COC is WHO 1, i.e. no restriction in use.*

Clinical implications

Women are advised not to conceive
  for 6 months after hCG levels are normal, and
  for at least 12 months from conclusion of any chemotherapy (risk of recurrent disease and teratogenic effects of the chemotherapy).

So what contraception should be used?
  Fortunately, while hCG levels are >5000IU/L ovulation is very improbable so barrier methods should be effective, and these are first choice for what is usually a short time.
  The progestogen-only methods are all now WHO 3 while hCG is elevated, and emergency contraception (EC) is also permitted (WHO 3).
  Combined hormonal methods can be used as soon as hCG concentrations are normal.
  Intrauterine methods are not recommended (WHO 4) until a normal menstrual cycle is established.

• If frank cancer is diagnosed, with chemotherapy in progress, avoid IUDs except with special approval from the regional centre: a progestogen-only method would often be best.

In summary, after the all-clear with respect to hCG monitoring has been given by the regional centre, any hormonal or intra-uterine method is usable (WHO 1).

Carcinomas of the ovary and of the endometrium
• Both are definitely less frequent in COC users.

A protective effect can be detected in ex-users for up to 15yrs, indeed for carcinoma of the ovary if lasts over 30 years. In both cases the risk is about halved among women who use COCs for 15 years. Suppression in COC users of ovulation and of normal mitotic activity in the endometrium are the accepted explanations of these findings.

Clinical implications: it would be reasonable for a woman known to be predisposed to either of these cancers to choose to use the COC primarily for this protective effect.

Colorectal cancer
There are very suggestive data from a number of studies that the pill also *protects* against this cancer.

Women who are apparently cured by local surgery for neoplasia of the ovary, cervix, and for malignant melanoma may all use COCs. The 'bottom line' when counselling COC takers is as follows: *Populations using the pill may develop different benign or malignant neoplasms from control populations, but it does not appear from computer modelling studies that the overall risk of neoplasia is increased.* See Fig. 22.1.

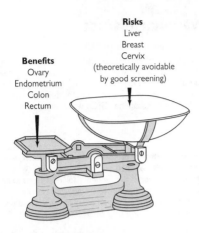

Fig. 22.1 Cancer and the pill: a balance.

Based on figure from *The Pill*, part of the Facts series. 6th edition. By permission of Oxford University Press.

Cardiovascular disease

Venous thromboembolism (VTE)

The UK 'pill-scare' in 1995 could have been minimized if the data had been presented as a *reduction* in VTE risk for women using levonorgestrel (LNG) or norethisterone (NET) pills: the *different* progestogens are really LNG and to a lesser extent NET, not the 'third-generation' progestogens desogestrel (DSG) and gestodene (GSD) which were adversely highlighted at the time.

Levonorgestrel (LNG):
- Opposes any estrogen-mediated rise in sex hormone-binding globulin (SHBG) and in high-density lipoprotein (HDL) cholesterol—and can even lower the latter if enough is given.
- Somatically, it also opposes the tendency for oestrogen to improve acne.
- LNG when combined with ethinylestradiol (EE) reduces the pro-coagulant effects of the latter on acquired activated protein-C resistance and the reduction of protein-S levels.

Norgestimate, the progestogen used in Cilest® and Evra®, the contraceptive patch, is in part metabolized to LNG. Yet both these two combination products with EE are more oestrogen-dominant than Microgynon 30®.

Any beneficial effect of LNG (and norethisterone (NET) and its pro-drugs) on VTE risk may not be as great as the epidemiology of 1995–1996 suggested. This is because of the well-established influence of prescriber bias and the 'healthy user' effect (which led, at the time of the studies, to women at lower intrinsic risk being more likely to be using the older LNG or NET pills—because the women with risk factors such as smoking and high BMI had been switched to what were thought to be the 'safer' newer products!).

Clinical implications Advice from the UK Department of Health (DoH) 'found no new safety concerns' about third-generation DSG or GSD products, and went on:

The spontaneous incidence of VTE in healthy non-pregnant women (not taking any oral contraceptive) is about 5 cases per 100 000 women per year. The incidence in users of second generation Pills is about 15 per 100 000 women per year of use. The incidence in users of third generation Pills is about 25 cases per 100 000 women per year of use: this excess incidence has not been satisfactorily explained by bias or confounding. The level of all of these risks of VTE increases with age and is likely to be increased in women with other known risk factors for VTE such as obesity.

Women must be fully informed of these very small risks ... Provided they are, the type of Pill is for the woman together with her doctor or other family planning professionals jointly to decide in the light of her individual medical history. [Author's emphasis]
- Using the incidence rates given by the DoH above, each year there will be 100 fewer cases of VTE per million users of an LNG product such as Microgynon30® (Schering Health Care) than among a similar number of women using a more oestrogen-dominant product. Using

an estimate of 2% for VTE mortality in the UK, this means a 2 per million greater annual VTE mortality for such a product than say Microgynon 30®. From Fig. 22.2, this risk difference is the same as that from 2h of driving.

- Hence, if a woman chooses to control a symptom such as acne by switching away from Microgynon 30® to an oestrogen-dominant product, all she needs to do is avoid one 2h drive in the whole of the next year to remain, in terms of VTE risk, effectively still on the Microgynon 30®!
- The risk difference is tiny but probably real—and therefore worth avoiding by the current UK policy of generally using an LNG product as first line, while being fully prepared to switch for symptom control upon request.
- The primary reason for choosing, or changing to, a more oestrogenic product, such as one containing DSG or GSD as the progestogen, is for the control of side-effects occurring on an LNG or NET product.

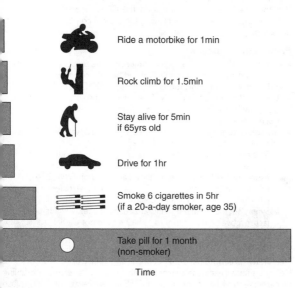

Ride a motorbike for 1min

Rock climb for 1.5min

Stay alive for 5min
if 65yrs old

Drive for 1hr

Smoke 6 cigarettes in 5hr
(if a 20-a-day smoker, age 35)

Take pill for 1 month
(non-smoker)

Time

Fig. 22.2 Time required to have a one in a million risk of death.
Adapted from Minerva, *British Medical Journal* (1988) and from *Pharmacoepidemiology* 1994).

Reproduced from *The Pill* part of the Facts series. 6th edition. By permission of Oxford University Press.

Arterial diseases: acute myocardial infarction (AMI), haemorrhagic stroke (HS) and ischaemic stroke (IS)

Acute myocardial infarction (AMI). If current or past pill-takers are *non* smokers studies find a nil or extremely small added risk of AMI.

Haemorrhagic stroke (HS), including subarachnoid haemorrhage. No increased risk due to the COC under age 35 unless there is also a risk factor such a hypertension (odds ratio (OR) 10) or smoking (OR 3). The risk increases with age, and this effect is magnified by current COC use, but with no effec of past use or long-duration use.

Ischaemic stroke (IS). Here there is a detectable increase in the OR due to pill taking in the range of 1.5 to a maximum of 2. Much of this risk seems to be focused within the subpopulation who suffer from migraine with aura (see below). The OR for hypertension is 3, and for smoking also 3.

Effect of dose/type of hormone It is believed, though never proven, that the modern low oestrogen pills help to minimize the arterial risks Whether the type of progestogen in the COC separately affects (as i can only do in those with risk factors) the arterial conditions above is still uncertain.

Prescribing guidelines

- Prescribers should always take a comprehensive personal and family history and check the woman's BMI and her BP to exclude **absolute and relative contraindications** to the use of COCs (see 📖 p. 305).
- A personal history of definite VTE remains an absolute contraindication to any hormonal method containing EE, combined with any progestogen.
- The risk factors for risk of future VTE and arterial wall disease must be assessed (see Tables 22.3 and 22.4):
  - Smoking is an independent risk factor for VTE, as well as arterial disease
  - Alone, one risk factor from either Table 22.3 or Table 22.4 is a relative contraindication (WHO 2 or 3 columns), unless it is particularly severe (WHO 4 column)
  - Synergism means that if WHO 3 already applies, any additional risk factor moves the category to WHO 4 ('Do not use')
  - Generally, however, COC use is acceptable on a WHO 3 basis when two WHO 2 factors apply.

Hereditary predispositions to VTE (thrombophilias) Almost the only indication for screening is a strong family history of one or more sibling or parents having had a spontaneous VTE under the age of 45. This justi fies testing for the genetic predispositions, including Factor V Leiden (the genetic cause of activated protein-C resistance) which, if identified, is classified as WHO 4. Even if all the results are normal, however, the COC remains WHO 2. The woman's strong family history cannot be discounted, since by no means all the predisposing abnormalities of the complex haemostatic system have yet been characterized.

Table 22.3 Risk factors for venous thrombo-embolism (VTE)

Risk factor	Absolute contraindication	Relative contraindication		Remarks
	WHO 4	WHO 3	WHO 2	
Personal or Family history (Fh) of thrombophilias, or of venous thrombosis in sibling or parent	Past VTE event; or identified clotting abnormality in this person, whether hereditary or acquired FH of a defined thrombophilia or *idiopathic* thrombotic event in parent or sibling <45 and thrombophilia screen not (yet) available	FH of thrombosis in parent or sibling <45 with recognized precipitating factor (e.g. major surgery postpartum) and thrombophilia screen not available	FH of thrombotic event in parent or sibling <45 with or without a recognized precipitating factor and *normal* thrombophilia screen FH in parent or sibling ≥45 or FH in second-degree relative [classified WHO 2 but tests not indicated]	*Idiopathic* VTE in a parent or sibling <45 is an indication for a thrombophilia screen if available. The decision to undertake screening in other situations (including where there was a recognized precipitating factor) will be unusual because very cost-ineffective—might be done on clinical grounds, in discussion with the woman Even a normal thrombophilia screen cannot be entirely reassuring, as some predispositions not yet known
Overweight—high Body Mass Index	BMI ≥ 40	BMI 30–39	BMI 25–29	See Note 5. below.
Immobility	Bed-bound, with or without major surgery; or leg fractured and immobilized	Wheelchair life, debilitating illness	Reduced mobility for other reason	Minor surgery such as laparoscopic sterilization is WHO 1

Table 22.3 (Contd.)

Varicose veins (VVs)	Current superficial vein thrombosis in the upper thigh Current sclerotherapy for VVs (or imminent VV surgery)	History of superficial vein thrombosis (SVT) in the lower limbs, no deep vein thrombosis	SVT does not result in pulmonary embolism, although this past history means some caution (WHO 2) in case it might be a marker of future VTE risk. Uncomplicated VVs are irrelevant to VTE risk (WHO 1)
Cigarette smoking	≥15 cigarettes per day	< 15 cigarettes per day	On balance the literature suggests a VTE risk from smoking, though less than the arterial disease risk it causes
Age >35	>51	35–51 if age is sole risk factor	

[1] A single risk factor in the relative contraindication columns indicates use of LNG/NET pill, if any COC used (as in BNF).

[2] Beware of synergism: more than one factor in either of relative contraindication columns. As a working rule, two WHO 2 conditions makes WHO 3; and if WHO applies (e.g. BMI 30–39) addition of either a WHO 3 or WHO 2 (e.g. reduced mobility) condition normally means WHO 4 (do not use).

[3] Acquired (non-hereditary) predispositions include positive results for anti-phospholipid antibodies—definitely WHO 4 since they also increase the risk of arterial events (Table 22.4)

[4] There are also important acute VTE risk factors, which need to be considered in individual cases: notably
• dehydration through any cause.
• long-haul flights and
• major and all leg surgery.

[5] There are minor differences in the above table from UKMEC, notably the author's more cautious categorization of BMIs >25.

Acquired predispositions to VTE (thrombophilias) Antiphospholipid antibodies which increase both VTE and arterial disease risk (Table 22.4,
Note 4) may appear in a number of connective tissue disorders, most
commonly in systemic lupus erythematosus (SLE). If identified, they absolutely contraindicate COC use (WHO 4).

Which pills are the current 'best buys' for women?

- *First-time users:* a low-dose LNG or NET product should remain the
  usual first choice. This is in part because first-timers will include an
  unknown subgroup who are VTE predisposed, VTE being a more
  relevant consideration than arterial disease at this age, and the pills
  suit the majority and cost less.
- *In the presence of a single WHO 2 or 3 risk factor for venous thrombosis:*
  the Summary of Product Characteristics (SPCs) for COCs state that
  DSG/GSD products are contraindicated.
  - This policy has merit if the COC is to be used solely *for
    contraception.* But
  - if there is a clear *therapeutic indication* for the COC, such as the
    polycystic ovarian syndrome (PCOS) with moderately severe acne,
    a different risk–benefit balance may apply. Extra therapeutic
    benefits from a more oestrogenic product may be judged to
    outweigh any expected extra risks—on a WHO 3 basis—because,
    for example, the woman has a BMI of 32. Relevant choices might
    be Marvelon®, Yasmin® or Dianette®. These probably all share the
    same (oestrogen-dominant) category—but only because they *lack*
    LNG: with its antagonizing EE effect.
  - Women with a single *definite arterial risk factor* (Table 22.4),
    e.g. *smokers, diabetics*—after a number of years VTE-free use *or* if
    the COC is used at all by *healthy women above the age of 35.* There
    is some suggestive evidence that DSG/GSD pills might have relative
    advantages for arterial wall disease. Therefore, for such *higher risk
    women,* or older women aged 35, using a 20mcg DSG or GSD
    product might be (at least) discussed. Any advantages in so doing
    are far from established, and changing to a different method
    altogether would usually be a better course. In the UK, Femodette®
    (GSD) or Mercilon® (DSG) are the relevant 20mcg EE products.
    Loestrin 20® would also be acceptable, and preferable if there
    were any WHO 3-level concern about VTE risk, since it contains
    a NET-group progestogen.

Table 22.4 Risk factors for arterial disease

Risk factor	Absolute contraindication	Relative contraindication		Remarks
		WHO 4	WHO 3	
Family history (FH) of atherogenic lipid disorder or of arterial CVS event in sibling or parent	Identified familial hyperlipidaemia in this person, persisting despite treatment	FH of known familial lipid disorder or *idiopathic* arterial event in parent or sibling <45 and client's lipid screening result: • not available or • confirmed and responding to treatment	Client has the less problematic common hyper-lipidaemia and responding well to treatment FH of arterial event with risk factor (e.g. smoking), in parent or sibling < 45, and lipid screen not available	FH of premature (<45) arterial CVS disease without other risk factors, or a known atherogenic lipid disorder in a parent or sibling, are indications for fasting lipid screen, if available (then check with laboratory re clinical implication of abnormal results) Despite any FH, normal lipid screen in client is reassuring, means WHO 1 (in contrast to thrombophilia screening)
Cigarette smoking	≥40 cigarettes/day	15–39 cigarettes/day	<15 cigarettes/day	Cut-offs here are somewhat arbitrary
Diabetes mellitus (DM)	Severe, longstanding or DM complications (e.g. retinopathy, renal damage, arterial disease)	Not severe/labile and no complications, young patient with short duration of DM		DM is always at least WHO 3 for the COC (safer options available)

Hypertension (consistently elevated BP, with properly taken BP measurements)	Systolic BP ≥160mmHg Diastolic BP ≥95mmHg	Systolic BP in range >140–159mmHg Diastolic BP >90 to 95mmHg On treatment for essential hypertension, with good control	BP regularly at upper limit of normal (i.e. near to 140/90mmHg) Past history of pre-eclampsia (WHO 3 if also a smoker)	Levels for WHO 4 and WHO 3 are consistent with UKMEC
Overweight, high BMI	BMI ≥ 40	BMI 30–39	BMI 25–29	High BMI increases arterial as well as VTE risk
Migraine	Migraine with aura Migraine without aura if attacks last >72h + no overuse of medication	Migraine without aura plus a strong added arterial risk factor	Migraine without aura	Relates to *thrombotic* stroke risk Triptan treatment does not affect the category
Age >35	>35 if a continuing smoker Age >51 for all others, even if risk-factor-free	35–51, if ex-smoker	Age 35–51 if free of all risk factors (yet even safer options are available)	In all persistent smokers, age >35 best classified as WHO 4. In ex-smokers, WHO 3 is because arterial wall damage may persist; but UKMEC permits WHO 2 after one year of not smoking

Notes

[1] Beware of synergism: more than one factor in either of relative contraindication columns. As a working rule, two WHO 2 conditions makes WHO 3; and if WHO 3 applies, (e.g. smoking >15 per day) addition of either a WHO 3 or WHO 2 (e.g. age 35) condition normally means WHO 4 (as in Table 22.3).

[2] The Pill seems to have a negligible, though not nil, adverse effect in arterial disease unless there is a risk factor. In continuing smokers, COC is generally stopped at age 35, in the UK.

[3] WHO numbers also relate to use for contraception: use of COCs for medical indications such as PCOS often entails a different risk–benefit analysis, i.e. the extra therapeutic benefits might outweigh expected extra risks.

[4] There are minor differences in the Table from UKMEC, notably the author's more cautious categorization with respect to smoking, hyperlipidaemia and DM.

Eligibility criteria for COCs

Absolute contraindications to COCs or other combined methods (e.g. Evra)

1. Past or present circulatory disease

- Any past proven arterial or venous thrombosis.
- Ischaemic heart disease or angina or coronary arteritis (Kawasaki disease—this is WHO 3 after recovery).
- Severe or combined risk factors for venous or arterial disease (see Tables 22.3 and 22.4) can be WHO 4—though usually graded lower (as below).
- Atherogenic lipid disorders (take advice from an expert, as indicated).
- Known pro-thrombotic states
  - abnormality of coagulation/fibrinolysis, i.e. congenital or acquired thrombophilias;
  - from at least 2 (preferably 4) weeks before until 2 weeks after mobilization following elective major or leg surgery (do not demand that the COC be stopped for minor surgery such as laparoscopy); during leg immobilization (e.g. after fracture) or varicose vein treatment; and
  - when going to high altitudes if there are added risk factors (otherwise WHO 3, see below).
- Migraine with aura (described on 📖 p. 314).
- Definite aura *without* a headache following.
- Transient ischaemic attacks.
- Past cerebral haemorrhage.
- Pulmonary hypertension, any cause.
- Structural (uncorrected) heart disease such as valvular heart disease or shunts/septal defects are only WHO 4 if there is an added arterial or venous thrombo-embolic risk (persisting, if there has been surgery). Always discuss this with the cardiologist—could be WHO 3, especially if patient always on warfarin. Important WHO 4 examples are:
  - atrial fibrillation or flutter whether sustained or paroxysmal—or not current but high risk (e.g. mitral stenosis);
  - dilated left atrium (>4cm);
  - cyanotic heart disease;
  - any dilated cardiomyopathy, but not a past history of any type when in full remission (WHO 2).
- In other structural heart conditions, if there is little or no direct or indirect risk of thromboembolism (this being the crucial point to check with the cardiologist), the COC is usable (WHO 3 or 2).

2. Disease of the liver

- Active liver cell disease (whenever liver function tests currently abnormal, including infiltrations and cirrhosis)
  - past pill-related cholestatic jaundice (if in pregnancy can be WHO 3)
  - Dubin–Johnson and Rotor syndromes (Gilbert's disease is WHO 2)
  - following viral hepatitis or other liver cell damage: but COCs may be resumed 3 months after liver function tests have become normal.

- Liver adenoma, carcinoma.
- Acute hepatic porphyrias; other porphyrias are usually WHO 3, but a non-steroid hormone method usually preferable.

3. History of serious condition affected by sex steroids or related to previous COC use

- SLE—also VTE risk.
- COC-induced hypertension.
- Pancreatitis due to hypertriglyceridaemia.
- Pemphigoid gestationis.
- Chorea.
- Stevens–Johnson syndrome (erythema multiforme), if COC associated.
- Trophoblastic disease but only until hCG levels are undetectable.
- Haemolytic uraemic syndrome (HUS) and thrombotic thrombocytopenic purpura (TTP). HUS in the past with complete recovery is generally WHO 2.

4. Pregnancy

5. Undiagnosed genital tract bleeding

6. Oestrogen-dependent neoplasms

- Breast cancer.
- Past breast biopsy showing premalignant epithelial atypia.

7. Miscellaneous

- Allergy to any pill constituent.
- Past benign intracranial hypertension.
- Specific to Yasmin®: because of the unique spironolactone-like effects of the contained progestogen drospirenone (DSP), this particular brand should be avoided—should any COCs be appropriate—in anyone at risk of high potassium levels (including severe renal insufficiency, hepatic dysfunction and treatment with potassium-sparing diuretics).

8. Woman's anxiety about COC safety unrelieved by counselling

Note that several of the above (e.g. 4–5, 8) are not necessarily permanent contraindications. Moreover, many women over the years have been unnecessarily deprived of COCs for reasons now shown to have no link, such as thrush; or which would have positively benefited from the method, such as 2° amenorrhoea with hypo-oestrogenism.

Relative contraindications to COCs

Unless otherwise stated, relative contraindications to COCs are WHO 2

- Risk factors for arterial or venous disease (see Tables 22.3 and 22.4). These are WHO 2, sometimes 3, provided that only one is present and that not of such severity as to justify WHO 4.
  - HUS (see above) in past history may be WHO 2 if complete recovery and not pill-associated (e.g. past *E. coli* 0157 infection as established cause of HUS).
  - Diabetes (minimum category being WHO 3), hypertensive disease and migraine all deserve separate discussion, below.
- Risk of altitude illness. This is not more probable because a climber is on COC; but, if it occurs, in its most severe forms there may be venous or arterial thromboembolism or patchy pulmonary hypertension, either of which would contraindicate the method. Hence all women travelling to above 2500m should be informed that the COC might increase the thrombotic component of severe arterial illness if that were to occur. For more details, see Barry and Pollard[1].
- Sex steroid-dependent cancer in prolonged remission (WHO 3); prolonged is defined as after 5 years by WHOMEC.
  - Prime example is breast cancer.
  - Malignant melanoma any time postdiagnosis is WHO 2 for the pill.
- If a young (<40yrs of age), first-degree relative has breast cancer (WHO 2).
- Established BBD.
- During the monitoring of *abnormal cervical smears* (WHO 2).
- During and after definitive *treatment for CIN* (WHO 2).
- Oligo-/amenorrhoea (COCs may be prescribed, after investigation—may be WHO 1, use unrestricted, if the purpose is to supply oestrogen in a woman needing contraception or to control the symptoms of PCOS).
- Hyperprolactinaemia (WHO 3, but only for patients who are on specialist drug treatment and with close supervision).
- Most chronic congenital or acquired systemic diseases (see below) are WHO 2:
  - sickle cell trait is WHO 1 but homozygous sickle cell disease is WHO 2 (though DMPA is preferred for this)
  - inflammatory bowel disease WHO 2, or 3 if severe because of VTE risk in exacerbations
  - otosclerosis (WHO 2)
  - gallstones (WHO 3, but WHO 2 after cholecystectomy)
  - very severe depression, if clear history of it being exacerbated by COCs (but unwanted pregnancies can be very depressing!).
- Diseases that require long-term treatment with enzyme-inducing drugs are WHO 3 (COC usable, see below, but alternative contraception preferred.

Alternatives to the COCs in these cases would be POP or barrier methods.

---

[1] Barry PW, Pollard AJ. Altitude illness. *BMJ* 2003; **326**: 915–919.

Diabetes mellitus (DM)

Consider as a WHO 3 condition even when there is no *known* diabetic tissue damage (cf. WHOMEC which classes well-controlled DM as WHO 2).

Clinically, given the high arterial disease risk, in particular, the POP (often Cerazette®) or Implanon® are definitely preferred alternatives.

Mercilon®, Femodette® or Loestrin 20® (see above) are COC options, but for limited duration and under careful supervision: for cases where there is no known arteriopathy, retinopathy, neuropathy or renal damage, nor any added arterial risk factor such as obesity or smoking—all of which mean WHO 4—and preferably if the duration of the disease has been short (Table 22.4).

Hypertension

- In most women on COCs there is a slight increase in both systolic and diastolic blood pressure (BP) within the normotensive range: ~1% become clinically hypertensive, and the rate increases with age and duration of use. If BP is repeatedly >160/>95 mmHg the method should be stopped; and if it then normalizes this pill-induced hypertension is WHO 4 for the future.
- Past severe toxaemia (pregnancy-induced hypertension) does not predispose to hypertension during COC use, but it is a risk factor for myocardial infarction (WHO 2), markedly so if the women also smokes (WHO 3).
- Essential hypertension (not COC related), when well controlled on drugs, is WHO 3, i.e. the COC is usable but not preferred.

Migraine

Migraines can be defined by the answers to the following questions:

'During the last 3 months did you have the following with your headaches?

1. You felt *nauseated* or sick in your stomach.

2. You were *bothered by light* a lot more than when you don't have headache.

3. Your headaches *limited your ability* to work, study or do what you needed to do for at least 1 day'.

Two 'yes' answers out of the three means the diagnosis of migraine.

Migraine and stroke risk

- Studies have shown an increased risk of ischaemic stroke in migraine sufferers and in COC users, and if combined there is 'summation' of risk.
- There is good evidence of exacerbation of risk by arterial risk factors, including smoking and increasing age above 35yrs.
- The presence of aura before or even without the headache is the main marker of risk (WHO 4), indeed not only for ischaemic stroke but also for coronary artery disease and myocardial infarction. It seems increasingly likely that there is no significantly increased risk through having migraine without aura, though for the present this is still classified as WHO 2. Given that the one year prevalence of any

migraine in women has been shown to be as high as 18%, it is crucial to identify the important subgroup with aura (1yr prevalence ~5%).

Migraine with aura

- Taking this crucial history starts by establishing the timing: *neurological symptoms of aura begin before the headache itself*, and typically last ~20–30min, max 60min, and stop before the headache (which may be very mild). Headache may start as aura is resolving or there may be a gap of up to 1h.
- Visual symptoms occur in 99% of true auras and hence should be asked about first.
- These are typically bright and affect part of the *field* of vision, on the same side in both eyes (homonymous hemianopia).
- Fortification spectra are often described, typically a bright scintillating zig-zag line gradually enlarging from a bright centre on one side, to form a convex C-shape surrounding the area of lost vision (which is a bright scotoma).
- Sensory symptoms are confirmatory of aura, occurring in around one-third of cases and rarely in the absence of visual aura; typically paraesthesia spreading up one arm or one side of the face or the tongue. The leg is rarely affected. They are positive symptoms, *not loss* of function.
- Disturbance of speech may also occur, in the form of nominal dysphasia.

Clinical implications—taking an aura history

- Ask the woman to describe a typical attack from the very beginning, including any symptoms before a headache. Listen to what she says *but at the same time watch her carefully.*
- A most useful **SIGN** that what she describes is likely to be true aura is if she draws something like a zig-zag line in the air with a finger to one or other side of her own head.

In summary, aura has three main features:

- Characteristic TIMING: onset BEFORE (headache) + duration ≤1h + Resolution before or with onset of headache.
- Symptoms VISUAL (99%).
- Description VISIBLE (using a hand).

Absolute contraindications (WHO 4) to starting or continuing the COC

- *Migraine with aura* or *aura without headache*. The *artificial oestrogen* of the COC is what needs to be avoided (or stopped) to minimize the additional risk of a thrombotic stroke.
- *Other migraines* (even without aura) which are *exceptionally severe* in a COC taker and last >72h despite optimal medication.
- *All migraines treated with ergot derivatives*, due to their vasoconstrictor actions.
- *Migraine without aura* **plus** multiple risk factors for arterial disease, or a relevant interacting disease (e.g. connective tissue diseases already linked with stroke risk).

NB: in all the above circumstances, any of the *progestogen-only*, i.e. *oestrogen-free*, hormonal methods may be offered immediately. Similar headaches may continue, but now without the potential added risk from prothrombotic effects of EE. Particularly useful choices are Cerazette®, Implanon®, the LNG-IUS or a modern copper IUD.

Migraine: relative contraindications for the COC

WHO 2, the COC is 'broadly usable' in the following cases:

- *Migraine without aura*, and also without an important arterial risk factor from Table 22.4 and still under the age of 35. NB: if these (or indeed other 'ordinary' headaches) occur only or mainly in the pill-free interval (PFI), tricycling the COC may help.
- *Use of a triptan drug* in the absence of an important other contraindicating factors.
- *The occurrence of a woman's first ever attack of migraine without aura* while on the COC. It is a reasonable precaution to stop the pill if she is seen during the attack. But after full evaluation of the symptoms—provided there were no features of aura or marked risk factors—the COC can be restarted later (WHO 2), with the usual counselling/caveats about future aura.

WHO 3. The COC is usable with caution and close supervision:

- **Primarily**, this is migraine without aura (common/simple migraine) with important risk factors for ischaemic stroke present (i.e. when WHO 3 anyway, the migraine without aura adds little further risk).
- **Secondly**, a clear past history of typical migraine *with aura* >5yrs earlier or only during pregnancy, with no recurrence, may be regarded as WHO 3. COCs may be given a trial, with counselling and regular supervision, along with a specific warning that the onset of definite aura (carefully explained) means that the user should:
  - stop the pill immediately
  - use alternative contraception and
  - seek medical advice as soon as possible.

Differential diagnoses

It may be difficult to distinguish such relatively common, migraine-associated transient ischaemia from rare organic episodes—true transient ischaemic attacks or TIAs (e.g. due to paradoxical embolism, which is an established risk of an atrial septal defect or persistent foramen ovale). TIAs are more sudden in onset than migraine aura and last over an hour, without other migraine symptoms such as nausea.

Upon suspicion these of course mean the same in practice, i.e. WHO 4, stop the pill immediately. But if an organic episode is a possibility, hospital investigation should also follow: including also for the following features which are not typical of migraine:

- focal epilepsy, severe acute vertigo, hemiparesis, ataxia, aphasia, unilateral tinnitus
- a severe unexplained drop attack or collapse
- monocular blindness (black scotoma), could rarely be a retinal vascular event or a symptom of TIA—amaurosis fugax
- progressive or persistent neurological symptoms (migraine is episodic with complete freedom from symptoms between attacks).

The pill-free interval (PFI)

There is evidence of return of significant pituitary and ovarian follicular activity during the PFI in about 20% of COC users. (See figure 22.3.)

- Renewed pill-taking after no more than a 7-day PFI restores ovarian quiescence. After 7 daily pills have been taken, missing more than 7 pills is likely to lead to breakthrough ovulation.

☞ Clinical implications

On the evidence available, WHO in the WHOSPR is now comfortable to define a 'missed pill' as one that is 24h late (not 12h, as hitherto) and has proposed two protocols based on the above pharmacology: one for up to 20mcg EE-containing products (recommended here for all formulations) and one for higher doses.

1. **'ONE tablet missed, for up to 24h'**: no special action needed, aside from taking the delayed pill and the next one on time.

 'ANYTHING MORE THAN ONE tablet missed': use CONDOMS as well, for the next 7 days.

Plus:

2. In the third active pill week, if any pill was completely (>24h) late, at the end of pack RUN ON to the next pack (skip 7 placebos if present).

Plus:

3. In the first pill week, EC is recommended IF—and only if—with sexual exposure since last pack, the COC user is a 'LATE RESTARTER' by >2 days or >2 pills are missed. This would be followed, next day, by recommencing pill taking with the appropriate day's tablet.

If 28-day packs are used (Microgynon ED®, which helps to avoid risky 'late' restarts), the user must learn which are the dummy 'reminder' tablets.

After pill-taking errors or severe vomiting, or short-term use of an enzyme inducer drug (see below), all women should be asked to report back if they have no withdrawal bleeding in the *next* PFI.

Vomiting and diarrhoea

If vomiting began >2h after a pill was taken, it can be assumed to have been absorbed. Otherwise follow 1–2–3 above, according to the number and timing of the tablets deemed to have been missed. Diarrhoea alone is not a problem, unless it is of cholera-like severity.

Previous combined pill failure

A woman who had a previous COC failure may claim perfect compliance or perhaps admit to omission of no more than one pill. She is likely to be a member of that one-fifth of the population whose ovaries show above average return to activity in the PFI. Such women may therefore be advised to take either three or four packets in a row (Fig. 22.4) followed by a shortened PFI. Both these regimens are often termed *tricycling*. The gap is shortened usually to 4 days, in high conception-risk cases, such as during the use of enzyme inducers (see below).

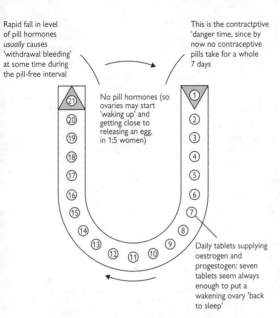

Rapid fall in level of pill hormones *usually* causes 'withdrawal bleeding' at some time during the pill-free interval

This is the contractptive 'danger time', since by now no contraceptive pills take for a whole 7 days

No pill hormones (so ovaries may start 'waking up' and getting close to releasing an egg, in 1:5 women)

Daily tablets supplying oestrogen and progestogen: seven tablets seem always enough to put a wakening ovary 'back to sleep'

Fig. 22.3 The pill cycle (21-day system).
Pill taking is drawn in a horseshoe for the important reason that a horseshoe is a symmetrical object. Hence, the pill-free interval can be lengthened, leading to the risk of conception, either side of the horseshoe, by forgetting (or vomiting) pills either at the beginning or at the end of the packet.

Reproduced from *The Pill* part of the Facts series. 6th edition. By permission of Oxford University Press.

Why have PFIs at all?

The pill-free week does promote a reassuring withdrawal bleed. If this is not seen as important, and to obtain certain other advantages, any woman may omit the PFIs and associated bleeds as a long-term *option*.

Seasonale is a dedicated packaging in the USA which provides four packets of the formulation of Microgynon®/Ovranette® in a row, followed by a 7-day, pill-free week, such that the user has a bleed every 3 months (i.e. seasonally!).

Clinical implications

In the short term, the gap between packets of monophasic brands is often omitted (upon request) to avoid a 'period' on special occasions. Users of phasic pills who wish to postpone withdrawal bleeds must use the final phase of a spare packet, or pills from an equivalent formulation, e.g. Norimin® in the case of TriNovum® or Microgynon 30® immediately after the last tablet of Logynon®.

Indications for a tricycling regimen (such as that shown in Fig. 22.4) using a monophasic pill.
- Woman's choice.
- Headaches, including migraine without aura—and other bothersome symptoms—if they occur regularly in the withdrawal week.
- Unacceptably heavy or painful withdrawal bleeds.
- Paradoxically, to help women who are concerned about absent withdrawal bleeds (less frequent pregnancy tests for reassurance!).
- Premenstrual syndrome—tricycling helps if COCs are used for this.
- Endometriosis, where after primary therapy a progestogen-dominant monophasic pill may be tricycled or, even better, given 365/365 for maintenance treatment.
- Epilepsy, which benefits from relatively more sustained levels of the administered hormones, and tricycling with a shortened PFI may also be indicated by the (enzyme-inducing) therapy given.
- Long term enzyme inducer therapy (discussed below).
- Wherever there is suspicion of decreased efficacy (see above).

In the last three instances (only), the PFI should be shortened to 4 days.

Breakthrough bleeding (BTB) may become a problem during tricycling, implying that the COC for that woman is unable to maintain endometrial stability for so long. One solution, provided a minimum of seven tablets have been taken since the last PFI (and it will usually be far more), is to advise at any time a definite 4–7 day break. Some women tolerate *bicycling* best, i.e. 42 days of continuous pill taking followed, depending on the indication, by a 4–7 day PFI.

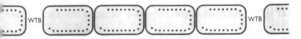

Fig 22.4 Tricycling (using four packs).

Note that they must be monophasic packs. The duration of the pill-free interval may also be shortened from 7 to 4 days (see text). WTB = withdrawal bleeds.

Reproduced from *The Pill* part of the Facts series. 6th edition. By permission of Oxford University Press.

Drug interactions

Drug interactions reduce the efficacy of COCs mainly by induction of liver enzymes, which leads to increased elimination of both oestrogen and progestogen (Fig. 22.5). Additionally, in a very small (but unknown) minority of women, disturbance by certain broad-spectrum antibiotics of the gut flora which normally split oestrogen metabolites that arrive in the bowel can reduce the reabsorption of reactivated oestrogen. According to WHOMEC, this effect is probably negligible clinically (but see below). It is certainly not a factor in the maintenance of progestogen levels and so is irrelevant to the POP. The most clinically important drugs with which interaction occurs are given in the lists below.

Enzyme inducer drugs (important examples) that interact with COCs

- Rifampicin, rifabutin.
- Griseofulvin (antifungal).
- Barbiturates.
- Phenytoin.
- Carbamazepine.
- Oxcarbazepine.
- Primidone.
- Topiramate (if daily dose >200mg).
- Modafinil.
- Some antiretrovirals (e.g. ritonavir, nevirapine)—full details are obtainable from www.hiv-druginteractions.org.
- St John's Wort—potency varies; CSM advises *non-use* along with COC.

Non-liver enzyme-inducing antibiotics that might possibly interact with COCs

On pragmatic and in part on medico-legal grounds, the UK Faculty of Family Planning and Reproductive Health Care (FFP&RHC) recommends that the short-term advice below be given for all such antibiotics—essentially all there are apart from rifampicin and rifabutin.[1]

In some cases this is overly cautious: co-trimoxazole, erythromycin and clarithromycin, for example, actually tend to raise blood levels of EE, although there is no evidence of thrombotic risk (grapefruit juice is similar!).

---

1 FFPRHC Guidance (April 2005). Drug interactions with hormonal contraception. *Journal of Family Planning and Reproductive Health Care* 2005; **31**: 139–151.

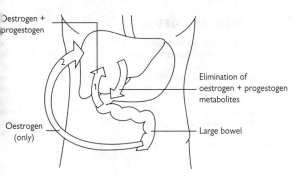

Fig. 22.5 The enterohepatic recirculation of oestrogen and its implications for drug interactions.
(1) First absorption of both hormones, via the liver. (2) Reabsorption of some oestrogen, but not progestogen. See text.

Other relevant drugs

- Note that none of the proton-pump inhibitors—including lansoprazole—is now regarded as having any clinically important enzyme induction effect.
- Ethosuximide, valproate and clonazepam, and most newer anti-epileptic drugs (including vigabatrin and lamotrigine), do not pose this problem.
- Lamotrigine levels can be *lowered* by COCs so starting a COC in a patient already taking this may result in poorer control of the epilepsy: a small increment in the dose of lamotrigine is all that is required. There is no problem in giving lamotrigine to patients already taking a COC, because the dose of lamotrigine is as usual titrated to the patient's needs.
- Ciclosporin levels can be *raised* by COC hormones: the risk of toxic effects means blood levels should be measured in sex steroid users.
- Drospirenone, the progestogen in Yasmin®, should not be used (WHO 4) in women on potassium-sparing diuretics (risk of hyper-kalaemia).

Clinical implications
Short-term use of any interacting drug (enzyme inducer or antibiotic)

Recommended regimen:
- Additional contraceptive precautions are advised during the treatment and
- should then be continued for a further 7 days.
- If at the end of treatment there are fewer than seven tablets left in the pack (i.e. third week), the next PFI should be eliminated (skip any placebo pills).
  - **Rifampicin** is such a powerful enzyme inducer that even if it is given only for 2 days (e.g. to eliminate carriage of meningococci), increased COC elimination by the liver must be assumed for 4 weeks thereafter, i.e. as though it had been given long term (see below). The extra contraception (e.g. condoms) should be continued to cover all that time therefore, plus *also* the elimination of any expected PFIs.

Long-term use of antibiotics

The large-bowel flora responsible for recycling oestrogens are reconstituted with resistant organisms within ~2 weeks. In practice, therefore, COCs are commenced in a woman who has been taking a tetracycline long term, there is no need to advise extra contraceptive precautions. There is a potential problem (now believed to involve very few women but clinically we never know which) in the reverse situation, i.e. when the tetracycline is first introduced to treat a long-term COC user. Even then:
- extra precautions need only be sustained for a maximum of 21 days (which includes the usual 7 days to restore full COC efficacy) with
- elimination of the next PFI if the 2 weeks of antibiotic use involved any of the last seven pills of a pack.

Long-term use of enzyme inducers

This applies chiefly to epileptic women and women being treated for tuberculosis. This is WHO 3, meaning that an alternative method of contraception is preferable—especially for those on rifampicin or rifabutin, whose adverse effects on efficacy of the COC are such that long-term users are strongly advised against it. Relevant options which should *always first be discussed* are the injectable, DMPA (with *no special advice* now needed to shorten the injection interval), an IUD or the LNG-IUS.

Recommended regimen

If the combined pill is nevertheless chosen, it is recommended:
- To prescribe an increased dose, usually 50–60 micrograms oestrogen by taking two tablets daily and also
- Advise one of the tricycle regimens described above. (This is particularly appropriate for epileptic women since the frequency of attacks is often reduced by the maintenance of steady hormone levels.)
- The PFI should also, logically, be shortened at the end of each tricycle: such that the next packet is started after 4 days, even if the withdrawal bleed has not stopped.

Only one 50 micrograms pill remains on the UK market (Table 22.5), and metabolic conversion of the pro-drug mestranol to EE is only ~75% efficient. Therefore, Norinyl-1® is almost identical to Norimin®. So the FFP&RHC recommends constructing a 50 or 60 micrograms regimen from two sub-50 micrograms products, e.g. two tablets daily of Microgynon 30®, or a Femodene® plus a Femodette® tablet. As this practice is unlicensed, this is named-patient use and the guidance should be followed.

Table 22.5 Formulations of currently marketed COCs

Pill type	Preparation	Oestrogen (micrograms)	Progestogen (micrograms)
Monophasic Ethinylestradiol/ norethisterone type	Loestrin 20®	20	1000 Norethisterone acetate*
	Loestrin 30®	30	1500 Norethisterone acetate*
	Brevinor®	35	500 Norethisterone
	Ovysmen®	35	500 Norethisterone
	Norimin®	35	1000 Norethisterone
Ethinylestradiol/ desogestrel	Microgynon 30 (also ED)®	30	150
	Ovranette®	30	150
Ethinylestradiol/ desogestrel	Mercilon® Marvelon®	20 30	150 150
Ethinylestradiol/ gestodene	Femodette®	20	75
Ethinylestradiol/ gestodene	Femodene (also ED)®	30	75
	Minulet®	30	75
Ethinylestradiol/ norgestimate	Cilest®	35	250
Ethinylestradiol/ drospirenone	Yasmin®	30	3000
Mestranol/ northisterone	Norinyl-1®	50	1000
Bi/triphasic Ethinylestradiol/ northisterone	BiNovum®	35 35	500 (7 tabs) 1000 } 833† (14 tabs)
	Synphase®	35 35 35	500 (7 tabs) 1000 } 714 (9 tabs) 500 (5 tabs)
	TriNovum®	35 35 35	500 (7 tabs) 750 } 750 (7 tabs) 1000 (7 tabs)
Ethinylestradiol/ levonorgestrel	Logynon (also ED)®	30 40 } 32† 30	50 (6 tabs) 75 } 92 (5 tabs) 125 (10 tabs)

Table 22.5 (Contd.)

	Trinordiol®	30 ⎫	50 ⎫	(6 tabs)
		40 ⎬32	75 ⎬92	(5 tabs)
		30 ⎭	125 ⎭	(10 tabs)
Ethinylestradiol/ gestodene	Tri-Minulet®	30 ⎫	50 ⎫	(6 tabs)
		40 ⎬32	70 ⎬79	(5 tabs)
		30 ⎭	100 ⎭	(10 tabs)
	Triadene®	30 ⎫	50 ⎫	(6 tabs)
		40 ⎬32	70 ⎬79	(5 tabs)
		30 ⎭	100 ⎭	(10 tabs)
Ethinylestradiol/ cyproterone acetate	Dianette‡®	35	2000	

* Converted to northisterone as the active metabolite.
† Equivalent daily doses for comparision with monophasic brands.
‡ Marketed primarily as acne therapy (see text)—and not intended to be used as a routine pill.
Other names in use worldwide are on website www.ippf.uk.
All preparation names are registered trade marks.

Note: there are some alternative formulations, as follows:

Femodette® is available as Sunya 20/75
Femodene®/Minulet® is available as Katya 30/75
Dianette® is available as Clairette 2000/35

Counselling and ongoing supervision

Starting the COC
- Full personal and family history.
- Individual teaching, backed by the FPA's user-friendly leaflet *Your Guide to the Combined Pill*.
- 21-day combined pill is started on either day 1 of the period without additional contraception, or less commonly on day 5 with the use of additional contraception for 7 days.
- In non-lactating women, 21-day or 28-day brands may be started 21 days after vaginal delivery provided there are no puerperal complications. Additional contraceptive measures should be taken for 7 days.
- After a first trimester termination, oral contraceptive can be started immediately (see Table 22.6).

Take-home messages for a new pill taker
- Your FPA leaflet: this is not to be read and thrown away; it is something to keep safely in a drawer somewhere, for ongoing reference.
- The pill only works if you take it correctly: if you do, each new pack will always start on the same day of the week.
- Even if bleeding, like a 'period', occurs (BTB), carry on pill taking—ring for advice if necessary. Nausea is another common early symptom. Both usually settle as your body gets used to the pill.
- *Never be a late restarter!* of your pill. Even if your 'period' (withdrawal bleed) has not stopped yet, never start your next packet late.
- Lovemaking during the 7 days after any packet is only safe if you do actually go on to the next pack. Otherwise, e.g. if you decide to stop the method, you must start using condoms after the last pill in the pack.
- For what to do if any pill(s) *are* >24h late, see above.
- Other things that may stop the pill from working include vomiting and some drugs (always mention that you are on the pill).
- See a doctor *at once* if any of the things on p. 332–3 occur, especially new headaches with strange *changes in your eyesight happening beforehand.*
- As a one-off, you can shorten one PFI to make sure all your future withdrawal bleeds avoid weekends.
- You can avoid bleeding on holidays, etc. by running packs together. (Discuss this with whoever provides your pills, if you want to continue missing out 'periods' long term.)
- Good though it is as a contraceptive, the pill does not give enough protection against *Chlamydia* and other STIs. Whenever in doubt, especially with a new partner, use a condom *as well.*

Table 22.6 Starting routines for COCs

Conditions before start	Start when?	Extra precautions for 7 days
1. Menstruating	On day 1 or 2 of period On day 3 or later Any time in cycle (Quick Start)	No* Yes Yes[†]
2. Postpartum (a) No lactation	Day 21 (low risk of thrombosis: first ovulations reported after day 28)	No
(b) Lactation	Not normally recommended (POP or injectable preferred)	
3. After induced abortion/ miscarriage	Same day or day 2 (day 21 if beyond 24 weeks gestation)	No
4. After trophoblastic tumour	One month after no hCG detected	As (1)
5. After higher dose COC	Instant switch After usual 7-day break	No Yes
6. After lower or same-dose COC	After usual 7-day break	No
7. After POP	First day of period	No
8. During POP-induced secondary amenorrhoea	Any day (end of packet)	No
9. Other secondary amenorrhoea including after DMPA (pregnancy excluded)[§]	Any day	Yes
10. First period after postcoital contraception	By day 2 when women sure her flow is normal or Quick Start[†], i.e. immediately	No Yes

* 28-day pill users also start with the first *active* pill on day 1. By applying the right sticky strip (out of seven supplied) for that weekday, all future pills are then labelled with the correct days.

[†] 'Quick Start' means starting any day provided the prescriber is satisfied there has been no significant earlier conception risk that cycle.

[‡] If usual 7-day break, rebound ovulation may occur at the time of transfer.

[§] Meaning prescriber is confident that no blastocyst or sperm is already in the upper genital tract, if necessary through a negative sensitive pregnancy test after at least 14 days of safe contraception or abstinence from intercourse.

Second choice of pill brand

Some women react unpredictably and it is a false expectation that any single pill will suit all women.

Bleeding side effects

Given the 'model' shown in Fig. 22.6 by the variability of blood levels and BTB risk, prescribers should try to identify the lowest dose for each woman which does not cause BTB. Even if BTB occurs, provided there is ongoing good compliance with pill taking, extra contraception (e.g. with condoms) does not need to be advised.

- The objective is that each woman should receive the least long-term metabolic impact that her uterus will allow, i.e. the lowest dose of contraceptive steroids that is just, but only just, above her bleeding threshold.

If BTB does occur and is unacceptable or persists beyond two cycles, a different or higher dose brand should be tried, though only **after** the checks in the 'D' check-list in the following box. Phasic COCs are generally second-choice formulations, but they are certainly worth trying here for BTB.

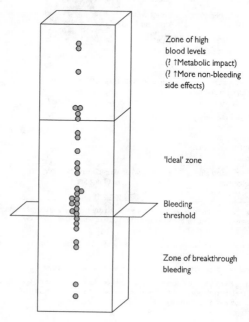

Zone of high blood levels
(? ↑Metabolic impact)
(? ↑More non-bleeding side effects)

'Ideal' zone

Bleeding threshold

Zone of breakthrough bleeding

Fig. 22.6 Schematic representation of the marked individual variation in blood levels of contraceptive steroids.

The following helpful check-list has been modified from Sapire[1].

Check-list for abnormal bleeding in a pill user

- **DISEASE** Consider examining the cervix (it is not unknown for bleeding from an invasive cancer to be wrongly attributed, and any bloodstained discharge should always trigger the thought '*Chlamydia?*').
- **DISORDERS of PREGNANCY** that cause bleeding (e.g. retained products if the COC was started after a recent termination of pregnancy).
- **DEFAULT** BTB may be triggered 2 or 3 days after missed pills and may be persistent thereafter.
- **DRUGS**, primarily enzyme inducers (see text). Cigarettes are also drugs in this context: BTB is statistically more common among smokers.
- **Diarrhoea** and/or **VOMITING** Diarrhoea alone has to be exceptionally severe to impair absorption significantly.
- **DISTURBANCES of ABSORPTION**, for example after massive gut resection.
- **DURATION of USE** too short, i.e. assessment is too early (minimal BTB which is tolerable for longer may then cease after 3 months use of any new formulation). The opposite possibility may apply during tricycling (see 📖 p. 318–9), namely that the duration of continuous use has been too long for that woman's endometrium to be sustained, in which case a *bleeding–triggered* 4–7 day break may be taken; or bicycling of two packets in a row may be substituted.
- **DOSE**, after the above have been excluded, it is possible to try a phasic pill if the woman is receiving monophasic treatment; increase the progestogen component (or oestrogen, if a 20 micrograms COC is in use); try a different progestogen.

Second choice if there are non-bleeding side effects

- When symptoms occur it is generally bad practice to give further prescriptions to control them without changing the COC—such as diuretics for weight gain or antidepressants for mood symptoms.
- There are two main preferred, if empirical, courses of action:
  - to decrease the dose of either hormone, if possible (in the limit, oestrogen can be eliminated by a trial of a POP); or
  - to change to a different progestogen.

[1] Sapire KE. Contraception and Sexuality in Health and Disease. New York: McGraw-Hill, 1990.

Which second choice of pill? Relative oestrogen excess

Symptoms
- Nausea.
- Dizziness.
- Cyclical weight gain (fluid), 'bloating'—Yasmin® is also worth a try here, given the anti-mineralocorticoid activity of DSP.
- Vaginal discharge (no infection).
- Some cases of breast enlargement/pain.
- Some cases of lost libido without depression, especially if taking an anti-androgen (Yasmin® or Dianette®).

Conditions
- Benign breast disease.
- Fibroids.
- Endometriosis.

Treat above with a relatively progestogen-dominant COC, such as Microgynon 30®. Loestrin 20® is an oestrogen-deficient option.

Which second choice of pill? Relative progestogen excess

Symptoms
- Dryness of vagina.
- Some cases of sustained weight gain—though there is actually no good evidence that modern COCs cause the weight gain for which they are often blamed.
- Depression/lassitude.
- Depressed mood ± associated loss of libido.
- Breast tenderness.

Conditions
- Acne/seborrhoea.
- Hirsutism.

Treat here with an oestrogen-dominant COC, such as Marvelon® or, in moderately severe cases of acne or hirsutism, Yasmin® or Dianette® (see text). (Caution is necessary, in that oestrogen dominance may correlate with a slightly higher risk of VTE, especially in, for example, obesity (Table 22.3)).

More about Yasmin®

Acne, seborrhoea and sometimes hirsutism may be benefited by any of the oestrogen-dominant COCs. Yasmin® is a monophasic COC containing 3mg DSP and 30 micrograms EE. DSP differs from other progestogens in COCs because:
- it acts as an anti-androgen, so the combination is an alternative to Dianette® for the treatment of moderately severe acne and the PCOS;
- it has diuretic properties due to anti-mineralocorticoid activity.

Yasmin® is welcomed as a new choice for appropriate women, for example:
- A clear indication for oestrogen/anti-androgen therapy, such as moderately severe acne.
- As a useful second choice for empirical control of minor side-effects: particularly those associated with fluid retention such as bloatedness and cyclical breast enlargement. It seems to be of value for women with the premenstrual syndrome, whether in their normal cycle or also occurring on another COC—in which case continuous use or tricycling is preferable.

Where does Dianette® feature now?

This is another anti-androgen plus oestrogen combination (CPA 2mg with EE 35 micrograms), licensed for the treatment of moderately severe acne and mild hirsutism in women. Dianette® is a reliable anovulant, usually giving good cycle control, and has similar rules for missed tablets, interactions, absolute and relative contraindications, and requirements for monitoring.

Duration of treatment with Dianette® needs to be individualized. In the SPC (data sheet), it is recommended that 'treatment is withdrawn when the acne or hirsutism is completely resolved', but 'repeat courses may be given if the condition recurs'. There are some concerns (not confirmed) related to hepatic effects, including of a greater benign and malignant liver tumour risk than other COCs in long-term use.

Clinically, therefore, there generally need to be good *therapeutic* indications to use Dianette® rather than Yasmin® (whose SPC mentions no particular duration limits). For those already taking the former, it is usual:
- To encourage patients to switch when their condition is controlled, perhaps after ~1yr, commonly to Marvelon®. The latter can be promoted to the woman as likely to be quite sufficient as *maintenance* treatment for what should now be much milder acne.
- If there is a relapse, try Yasmin®, or:
- exceptionally it may be appropriate to return to use of Dianette® for much longer.

Stopping COCs

- First menstruation after stopping COCs (for any reason) is often delayed by up to ~6–8 weeks.
- 2° amenorrhoea for 6 months should always be investigated, whether or not it occurs after stopping COCs—the link will be coincidental and not causal.
- If switching brands
  - 21 day to 21 day without break—contraception maintained
  - 21 day to 21 day with break—extra precautions advised for first 7 days of new brand unless latter is higher dose (📖 p. 327)
  - 28 day to 21 day—omit placebos and start new brand without break
  - From pill to patches: apply patch on first day of withdrawal bleed, no extra precautions are necessary.

Listed below are the (only) reasons for discontinuing COCs immediately or soon, and should be understood by all well-counselled women from their first visit. The worst implications of these symptoms are pill-related thrombotic or embolic catastrophes in the making, or onset of migraine with aura. Often there is another explanation and if so the COC may be recommended. The COC because of its contained EE should be stopped, but any progestogen-only method could be started immediately pending diagnosis.

Symptoms for which COCs should be stopped immediately, pending investigation and treatment

- Unusual or severe and very prolonged headache.
- Diagnosis of aura (see above), usually involving loss of part or whole of the field of vision on one side;
- Loss of sight in one eye (unrelated to migraine, see 📖 p. 315).
- Disturbance of speech (nominal dysphasia in migraine with aura).
- Numbness, severe paraesthesia or weakness on one side of the body, e.g. one arm, side of the tongue; indeed, any symptom suggesting cerebral ischaemia or TIA.
- A severe unexplained fainting attack or severe acute vertigo or ataxia.
- Focal epilepsy.
- Painful swelling in the calf.
- Pain in the chest, especially pleuritic pain.
- Breathlessness or cough with blood-stained sputum.
- Severe abdominal pain.
- Immobilization, e.g.
  - after most lower limb fractures or
  - *major* surgery or
  - leg surgery.

For all these, stop COC and consider heparin treatment. If an elective procedure is planned and the pill stopped >2 weeks ahead (4 weeks preferable), anticoagulation may be unnecessary. Good contraception can be maintained nowadays by switching to and then from Cerazette® which is believed to have negligible pro-thrombotic effects.

Other reasons for early discontinuation
- Acute jaundice.
- BP >160/>95mmHg (either figure) on repeated measurement.
- Severe skin rash (e.g. erythema multiforme).
- Detection of a significant new risk factor, e.g. onset of severe SLE, first diagnosis of breast cancer.

Pill follow-up

Primarily entails two items to be monitored:
- BP.
- Headaches, especially migraine.

Blood pressure

- Recorded before COCs are started and checked after 3 months (1 month in a high-risk case) and subsequently at intervals of 6 months.
- After a minimum of 15 months, if there is no rise between successive measurements, the interval can reasonably be increased to annually in women without risk factors (with a clear understanding that they may return for advice sooner, as desired).
- COCs should always be stopped altogether if BP exceeds 160/95 mmHg on repeated measurements.

Headaches

Not to ask about a COC-taker's headaches at the regular pill follow-up visit would be a serious omission.

Screening

Breast and bimanual pelvic examinations or monitoring blood tests have no relevance to pill follow-up.

Congenital abnormalities and fertility issues

- Even with exposure during organogenesis, meta-analyses of the major studies fail to show an increased risk. If present, it must be very small.
- Used *prior to* the conception cycle, there is no good evidence for any adverse effects on the fetus of COCs.

What about 'taking breaks' to optimize fertility?

These are of no value as there is no evidence that COCs can cause any permanent loss of fertility.

Summary

- The first visit for prescription of COCs is by far the most important and should never be rushed.
- The LARCs, long-term and 'forgettable' contraceptive options, should always be included in the discussion, despite the woman's presenting a request for what she happens to know about (most probably the pill).
- If the pill remains her choice, along with discussing the risks and benefits, and fully assessing her medical and family history, all at her level of understanding, there is much ground to cover (see Take-home messages list above). Often it is useful to share this between the doctor and practice or clinic nurse.
- Thereafter there are really only three key components to COC monitoring during follow-up:
  - BP.
  - Headaches.
  - Identification and management of any new risk factors/diseases/ side-effects.

Other combined methods

Transdermal combined hormonal contraception
Evra®

- A transdermal patch delivering EE with norelgestromin, the active metabolite of NGM.
- The daily skin dose of 150 micrograms norelgestromin and 20 micrograms EE produces blood levels in the reference range of those after a tablet of Cilest® but without either the latter's diurnal fluctuations or the oral peak dose given to the liver.
- All the absolute and relative contraindications and indeed most of the above practical management advice about the COCs apply.
- About 2% of women in the trials had local skin reactions which led to discontinuation. The patch has generally good adhesion even in hot climates and when bathing or showering; the incidence of detachment of patches was 1.8% (complete) and 2.9% (partial).
- In the pooled analysis of the RCT studies, the failure rate for consistent users of Evra® was similar to that of the oral pills, i.e. <1 per 100 woman-years.

Maintenance of efficacy of Evra®

- Due to evidence of a higher failure rate (and the VTE risks of likely high BMI), avoid use of Evra® at all if body weight is >90kg.
- Warn the user that the contraceptive is in the glue of the patch, so a dry patch that has fallen off should not be re-used!
- Each patch is worn for 7 days, for three consecutive weeks followed by a patch-free week.

Clinically, the patch is therefore a useful alternative to offer to those who find it difficult to remember a daily pill, especially as, if the patch user does forget, there is a 2-day margin for error for late patch change. However:

- As with the COC it is essential never to lengthen the contraception-free (patch-free) interval.
- If this interval *exceeds* 8 days for any reason (either through late application or the first new patch detaching and this being identified late), advise extra precautions for the duration of the first freshly applied patch (i.e. for 7 days). This should be after immediate emergency contraception if there has been sexual exposure during the preceding patch-free time.
- Absorption problems through vomiting/diarrhoea, and tetracycline by mouth, have no effect on this method's efficacy, but:
- During any short-term enzyme inducer therapy, and for 28 days after this ends, additional contraception, e.g. with condoms, is advised, plus elimination of any patch-free intervals during this time.

Transvaginal combined hormonal contraception

- NuvaRing® is a combined vaginal ring which releases etonogestrel (3-keto-desogestrel) 120 micrograms and EE 15 micrograms per day, thus equating to some degree with 'vaginal Mercilon®'.
- It is normally retained (though there is an unrestricted option to remove it for up to 3h during sexual activity) for 3 weeks and then taken out for a withdrawal bleed during the 4th.
- Pending more dedicated information, all the absolute and relative contraindications, and most of the above practical management advice about the COC, also apply to NuvaRing®.

Maintenance of efficacy of NuvaRing®

- Expulsions may be a problem for some (usually parous) women, primarily during the emptying of bowels or bladder, and therefore readily recognized.
- As with the COC, it will still be essential never to lengthen the contraception-free (ring-free) interval. If for any reason this exceeds 8 days, advise extra precautions for 7 days. As for Evra®, EC should be immediate if there has been sexual exposure during any ring-free time of >8 days.
- Absorption problems, vomiting/diarrhoea and broad-spectrum antibiotics have no effect on this method's efficacy.
- During any short-term enzyme inducer therapy, and for 28 days after this ends, additional contraception, e.g. with condoms, is advised, plus elimination of any ring-free intervals during this time.

Progestogen-only pill (POP)

Introduction

- five varieties of POP are available (Table 23.1)
- four of the old type which variably inhibit ovulation and
- the fifth, Cerazette®, a primarily anovulant product.

Unless otherwise stated the abbreviation POP will refer to the four old-type POPs.

Table 23.1 Available POPs

Product	Constituents	Course of treatment
Noriday®	350 micrograms norethisterone	28 tablets
Micronor®	350 micrograms norethisterone	28 tablets
Femulen®	500 micrograms etynodiol diacetate	28 tablets
Norgeston®	30 micrograms levonorgestrel	35 tablets
Cerazette®	75 micrograms desogestrel	28 tablets

Mechanism of action and maintenance of effectiveness

- Fertile ovulation is prevented in 50–60% of cycles.
- In the remainder there is reliance mainly on *progestogenic interference with mucus penetrability*. This 'barrier' effect is readily lost, so that each tablet daily must be taken within 3h of the same regular time.

Effectiveness

- Failure rate of 3.1 per 100 woman-years between the ages 25 and 29, but this improved to 1.0 at 35–39 years of age and was as low as 0.3 for women >40 years of age.

Effect of body mass (not BMI)

Studies are suggestive, but not conclusive, that the failure rate of old-type POPs may be higher with increasing weight. Pending more data, a logical policy now is to use Cerazette® as first choice for women >70kg (irrespective of height), especially if they are young.

Missed pills

After missing a POP for >3h (if Cerazette®, for >12h, see below) the woman should:

- take that day's pill immediately and the next one on time;
- use added precautions for the next 2 days.

If there has already been *intercourse without added protection between the time of first potential loss of the mucus effect and through to its restoration by 48h* then:

- Immediate EC with levonorgestrel (see below) is also advised, with the next POP taken on time.

What action is necessary during full lactation with ordinary POPs and in Cerazette® users (who have 12h of 'leeway' anyway)?

Here there is established anovulation. So only the first two bullets above would apply and EC would be unnecessary in most cases. Pending more data it could be given on a 'fail-safe' basis for omissions of more than one pill, i.e. beyond 24h.

More about lactation and the POP

According to LAM (see Fig. 19.2), even without the POP there is only ~2% conception risk if all three LAM criteria continue to apply, namely (to recap):

- amenorrhoea, since the lochia ceased;
- full lactation—the baby's nutrition effectively all from its mother;
- baby not yet 6 months old.

This is why on any POP during full lactation postcoital contraception would very rarely be indicated for missed POPs. But because breastfeeding varies in its intensity, if a tablet is 3h late it is still usual to advise additional precautions during the next two tablet-taking days.

What dose to the baby?

- During lactation, with all POPs including Cerazette®, the dose to the infant is believed to be harmless, but this aspect must always be discussed. The least amount of administered progestogen gets into the breast milk if an LNG POP is used. The quantity is the equivalent of one POP in 2 years, considerably less than the progesterone of cow's milk origin found in formula feeds.
- If EC is required (rather rarely, see above) by a breastfeeding mother, for just 24h she may wish to express and discard her breast milk, though even then there is no evidence that this higher LNG dose would cause her baby any harm.

Weaning

The margin for error in POP taking will diminish at weaning. If efficacy is at a premium, they should, for example, be given a supply of the COC or Cerazette® (unless that was already the POP being used in lactation) to start
- when breast milk stops being their baby's main nutrition, or
- no later than the first bleed.

Drug interactions

Broad-spectrum antibiotics do not interfere with the effectiveness of POPs or indeed any progestogen-only method.

Enzyme inducers Another highly effective contraceptive method is advised during use of liver enzyme inducers such as rifampicin or carbamazepine and, as necessary, for 4 weeks or more thereafter (see Chapter 22). Long-term treatment with enzyme inducers is WHO 3, but if a suitable alternative contraceptive is not identified and the couple do not wish to use condoms indefinitely, taking two tablets daily is an option (but unlicensed, 📖 p. 436).

Bosentan (an endothelin antagonist) is a particular enzyme inducer drug that would never be relevant for the COC, since it is used to treat pulmonary hypertension (which is WHO 4 for the COC). However, Cerazette® (see below) could be a very appropriate contraceptive for a young woman with this serious condition, in which pregnancy can be lethal: again, taking two tablets daily to compensate for the enzyme induction.

Risks and disadvantages

Being EE-free, these are exceptionally safe products. There are negligible changes to most metabolic variables. There is no proven causative link:
- with any tumour
- with venous or (less certainly) arterial disease,

Side-effects

- Main side-effect of POPs and Cerazette® is irregular bleeding.
- The irregularity can include *oligomenorrhoea*. FSH is not completely suppressed even during the amenorrhoea, which is mainly caused by LH suppression. There is therefore enough follicular activity at the ovary to maintain adequate mid-follicular phase oestrogen levels. Pending more data, this means there is *not* the concern about bone density reduction which persists for DMPA (see below).

The remaining relative contraindications, in which the POP method is generally WHO 2 and so may often be considered indications when alternatives are unsuitable are:

Relative contraindications (WHO 2) for POP and Cerazette® use

- Past VTE or severe risk factors for VTE—often an indication (see above).
- Risk factors for arterial disease; more than one risk factor can be present, in contrast to COCs.
- Current liver disorder—even if there is persistent biochemical change.
- Most other chronic severe systemic diseases (but WHO 3 if the condition causes significant malabsorption of sex steroids).
- Family history of breast cancer (WHOMEC says WHO 1).

Counselling and ongoing supervision

The starting routines are summarized in Table 23.2.

A crucial aspect of counselling is: how not to forget, given the 3h time window (and only 12h with Cerazette®). Mobile phone alarms and text messaging may be invaluable.

Frequent or prolonged menstrual bleeding

This is the main nuisance side-effect. With advance warning it may be tolerated. Improvement appears more likely with Cerazette®.

Amenorrhoea

Except during full lactation, prolonged spells of amenorrhoea occur most often in older women. Once pregnancy is excluded, the amenorrhoea must be the result of anovulation and so signifies very high efficacy.

Non-bleeding side-effects

These are rare with POPs, apart from the complaint of
- *Breast tenderness.* Though common this is usually transient; if it recurs it can sometimes be overcome by changing POPs—especially to Cerazette®.
- *Functional cysts* or luteinized unruptured follicles are also not uncommon; however, most are symptomless and pelvic pain on one or other side is relatively unusual.

Clinically, if they are symptomatic, functional cysts among POP users can lead to problems in the differential diagnosis from ectopic pregnancy (pain, menstrual disturbance and a tender adnexal mass being present in both conditions).

Monitoring

The BP of POP takers is checked initially, but, thereafter, if still normal at the 3-month follow-up visit, it really does not need to be checked more often than for other women. When raised during COC use, it usually reverts to normal on POPs.

Return of fertility after all POPs including Cerazette®

This is rapid: indeed clinically, from the user's point of view, fertility after stopping must be assumed to be immediate.

Menopause

Establishing ovarian failure at the menopause is less important than with the COC, since all the POPs are safe enough products to continue using well into the late 50s. Hence, first switching to any POP from the COC can be a reassuring way to manage that often difficult transition out of the reproductive years.

If there is amenorrhoea above the age of 50 on an old-type POP (not the pituitary-suppressing Cerazette®), a high blood FSH measurement (>30IU/L) suggests ovarian failure. Two high values 6 weeks apart, especially if there are vasomotor symptoms, would make the likelihood of a later ovulation very low. Should the FSH be found to be low, however, this suggests continuing ovarian function and, if the POP is not simply continued, the need for an additional contraceptive—such as condoms or, at this age, 'weaker' methods such as the sponge or spermicide.

Table 23.2 Starting routine for POPs

Condition before start	Start when?	Extra precautions
Menstruation	Day 1 of period	No
	Day 2 or later	7 days
	Any time in cycle ('Quick Start')	7 days[1]
Postpartum		
No lactation	Usually day 21	No
Lactation	Day 21—maybe later if 100% lactation	No
After induced abortion/miscarriage	Same day	No
After COCs	Instant switch	No
Amenorrhoea (e.g. postpartum)	Any time[2]	7 days

[1] Can start any day in selected cases if the prescriber is satisfied there has been no conception risk on the starting day.

[2] If prescriber is confident that no blastocyst or sperm is already in upper genital tract—see (📖 p. 430–1).

Cerazette®

Mechanism of action and maintenance of effectiveness
- This product contains 75 micrograms desogestrel; it blocks ovulation in 97% of cycles and had a failure rate in the premarketing study of only 0.17 per 100 woman-years (in 'perfect' users not also breastfeeding).
- 12h of 'leeway' in pill-taking have been approved before extra precautions are advised—these then being for 2 days, as for other POPs (though the manufacturer's SPC still recommends 7 days).
- Cerazette® shares the medical safety, rapid reversibility but also, unfortunately, the tendency to irregular bleeding side-effects and functional ovarian cyst formation of the old-type POPs.

Starting routines are unchanged from those in Table 23.2.

Advantages and indications
- Cerazette® is free of all the risks attributable to EE, plus no effects on BP have been reported.
- Cerazette® is a good option for many young fertile women with complicated structural heart disease or pulmonary hypertension (see above).
- Cerazette® is now the first-choice POP for a woman weighing >70kg unless she is breastfeeding or >45 years of age, in which case any POP would be effective.
- Cerazette® also usually ablates the menstrual cycle like COCs, but again without using EE. So it has potentially beneficial effects and can be tried in a range of menstrual disorders, especially:
  - dysmenorrhoea
  - menorrhagia
  - mittelschmerz
  - premenstrual syndrome (PMS)
  - Cerazette® may also be an alternative primarily anovulant method when there is a past history of ectopic pregnancy.

Problems and disadvantages
- Irregular bleeding remains a very real problem. Despite having a higher incidence of (more acceptable) amenorrhoea than with existing POPs, Cerazette® like other POPs and Implanon still appears to provide adequate follicular-phase levels of oestradiol (see above).

Contraindications
These, whether WHO 4, 3 or 2, are very similar to those for old-type POPs. The main difference is that Cerazette® is more effective, making it positively suitable for a past history of ectopic pregnancy.

In summary, Cerazette® may well become a first-line hormonal contraceptive for many women. However, there is no indication to use it rather than a cheaper old-type POP in lactation or in older women, especially in those >45 years of age.

Mechanism of action and effectiveness

- DMPA is one of the most effective among reversible methods (Table 1).
- 'Perfect use' failure rate of 0.3%, typical use 3% in the first year of use.
- It functions primarily by causing anovulation, with effects on the cervical mucus similar to the COC, as back-up.

Potential drug interactions

The liver ordinarily clears the blood, achieving complete clearance of the drug and—as enzyme inducers cannot increase clearance beyond 100%—there is no requirement to shorten the injection interval. This applies even to users of the most powerful enzyme inducers, rifampicin or rifabutin.

Starting routines

Timing of the first injection

- In menstruating women, the first injection should ideally be given on day 1 but can be up to day 5 of the cycle; if given later than day 5 (including *much* later if abstinence believably claimed to that day), advise 7 days extra precautions.
- If a woman is on a COC or POP or Cerazette® up to the day of injection, the injection can normally be given at any time, with no added precautions.
- Postpartum (when the woman is not breastfeeding) or after a second-trimester abortion, the first injection should normally be at about day 21 and, if later, with added precautions for 7 days. If later and still amenorrhoeic, pregnancy risk must be excluded. Earlier use can lead to prolonged heavy bleeding but is sometimes clinically justified,
- During lactation, if chosen, DMPA is best given at 6 weeks. Lactation is *not* inhibited and the dose to the infant is small and believed to be entirely harmless.
- After miscarriage or a first-trimester abortion, injection on the day (or after expulsion of fetus if a medical procedure). If the injection is given beyond the 7th day advise 7 days' extra precautions.

Overdue injections of DMPA with continuing sexual intercourse

Author's protocol (which is rather more cautions than UKMEC).
- From day 85 to 91 (13th week), injection plus condoms or equivalent to be used during the next 7 days.
- From day 92 to 98 (14th week), injection plus EC by hormone (or more rarely copper IUD) as appropriate, plus condoms for 7 days.
- Beyond day 98, end of 14th week.
  - The next injection is best postponed, usually for a few days.
  - If possible, agreement is reached with the woman that she will either abstain or use condoms with greater care than ever before, UNTIL there has been a total of 14 days since the last sexual exposure plus a sensitive pregnancy test is then negative.
  - If a sensitive (20–25IU/L) pregnancy test is then negative, the chances of a conception are negligible and the next dose can be given along with the usual advice for a further 7 days of added contraception, e.g. with condoms. No EC would then be needed, but a follow-up pregnancy test in a further 2 weeks might be wise.
- If the woman is not prepared to abstain or use condoms for the necessary days to reach 14 since her last sex, a useful compromise is to provide the POP for that time and then proceed as above. The teratogenic risks to a fetus exposed to the POP (and indeed DMPA) have been established as very low.

In all circumstances, counsel the woman regarding possible failure and the need for a check pregnancy test if there is doubt.

Indications

The main indications are

- the woman's desire for a highly effective method that is independent of intercourse and unaffected by enzyme inducers, and
- when other options are contraindicated or disliked.
- A past history of ectopic pregnancy or, like all other progestogen-only methods, of thrombosis (see earlier comments for the POP), e.g. for effective contraception while waiting for major or leg surgery (Cerazette® is another option here).

If it causes amenorrhoea, DMPA is positively beneficial in:

- endometriosis;
- past symptomatic functional cysts;
- other menstrual disorders.

Advantages

DMPA has
- obvious contraceptive benefits (effective, 'forgettable'), but the data imply that it also shares
- most of the non-contraceptive benefits of the COC described above, including protection against pelvic infection and endometrial cancer, while having
- even greater safety, with respect to mortality and serious morbidity, than the COC. This should strongly counterbalance any concerns about bone density, to be described below.

Problems and disadvantages

Metabolic changes are minimal, aside from some evidence of reduction in HDL cholesterol.

The main problems are
- Irregular, sometimes prolonged bleeding.
- Amenorrhoea and potential hypo-oestrogenism.
- Impossibility of reversal of the effect of a dose (for at least 3 months, sometimes longer). It is unfair not to mention this fact in advance.
- Delayed return of fertility—also something to warn about (see below).
- Weight gain (the latter can be marked in some cases).
- Some concern re reduced bone density—which is probably exaggerated.

Menstrual abnormalities

These are an obstacle to any large increase in the method's popularity.

In the management of *frequent or prolonged bleeding*
- First, always exclude a non-DMPA-related cause (on lines of 📖 p. 329).
- It has a better prognosis than with implants, being usually an early problem then generally followed by amenorrhoea after 3–6 months.
- If it does not resolve, the next injection may be given early (but not less than 4 weeks since the last dose). However:
- Clinical experience suggests that giving additional oestrogen is more successful, though not proven in trials. The rationale is to provide oestrogen cyclically to produce some 'pharmacological curettages', i.e. withdrawal bleeds designed to shed the existing endometrium that is bleeding in an unacceptable way—in the hope that a 'better' endometrium will be developed post-treatment. The plan should be explained to the woman, who should also understand that it is not guaranteed to work. The treatment options are:
  - 🔹 EE 30 micrograms (as such or more usually within a pill Microgynon 30). It is given daily for 21 days, usually for three cycles. Courses may be repeated if an acceptable bleeding pattern does not follow.
  - 🔹 If the woman has a WHO 3 or 4 contraindication to EE an alternative that was effective short-term (with Implanon®) is doxycycline 100mg bd for 5 days (benefit probably being additional to treating Chlamydial endometritis, if present, but test for this first).

Amenorrhoea occurs in most long-term users and is usually very acceptable after appropriate counselling.

Bone density

After >20 years of research but no RCTs nor adequate comparative studies, there remains uncertainty: not about the low follicular-phase estradiols that are indeed found in many DMPA users but about their implications for bone health.

We know that:

Mean bone density is lower in DMPA users than controls in cross-sectional comparisons, including among women above age 45. This finding is unconnected to the bleeding pattern (may or may not occur in women experiencing either amenorrhoea or irregular bleeding). It increases upon discontinuation (suggestive of a real effect; but also very reassuring for reversibility).

From limited evidence, there is decreased bone mineral density in adolescent DMPA users compared with controls using implants (or COCs). This has raised concern that *peak bone mass* that is fully developed by age 25 might be lower in users.

Yet:

Long-term DMPA-using women examined after their menopause and lifetime never users have *not* been shown to differ in their bone densities, suggesting recovery of bone mass after stopping.

An excess of limb or vertebral fractures has never been shown in long-term DMPA users.

Based on the above, WHOMEC therefore simply states that DMPA is WHO 2 for adolescents and for women over age 45. American and UK drug regulators have been more cautious, however; see below.

How long to use DMPA, in the UK?

The CSM circular (18 November 2004) had one main recommendation, namely *'careful re-evaluation of risks and benefits in all those who wish to continue use for more than 2 years'*

Clinically, in the UK, the following is now advised:

Protocol for the choice and duration of use of DMPA

If there is known osteopenia or strong risk factors exist, namely:
- Long-term corticosteroid treatment.
- $2°$ amenorrhoea, due to anorexia nervosa or marathon-running.
- a significant malabsorption syndrome.

For all these, DMPA is WHO 4, but the category could become WHO 3 if a bone scan shows no osteopenia, the risk factor has ceased and the young woman has been obtaining either natural oestrogen during normal cycling or EE through the COC.

- Under age 19, due to above concern that it may prevent achievement of peak bone mass, WHOMEC classifies DMPA as WHO 2; and the UK advice of November 2004 is similar, to use it first-line 'but **only** after other methods have been discussed' and are unsuitable or unacceptable.
- Above age 45. DMPA is also WHO 2 above age 45 (as by now possibility of incipient ovarian failure and gentler methods such as the POP are available which would be equally effective at this age).

For all other women
- DMPA remains a highly effective, safe and 'forgettable' method, usable by almost any woman in the childbearing years.
- In the UK it is now perceived as *very useful for fairly short-term use, after which switching to another long-term method such as an implant would be usual.*
- There should be a regular 'formal' 2-yearly discussion and reassessment of alternatives but *without blood tests or any imaging. Such (e.g. bone density scanning) would only be appropriate if indicated for that particular woman on specific clinical grounds.*
- Many will therefore choose to switch from DMPA to another long-acting method, e.g. to Implanon®, IUD or IUS, after 2, 4, 6 or 8yrs.
- But if the woman wishes to use DMPA for longer, even much longer, it is as always her right to decide to do so, on the 'informed user-chooser' basis, after counselling about the uncertainty.

Remember, when all is said and done, that DMPA is clearly safer than the EE-containing COC!

As it is recommended as an alternative in the protocol, are there not similar bone density concerns with long-term Implanon®?

No, the data are reassuring so far, re both oestradiol and bone density: in comparative 2yr studies both remained similar to those in copper IUD users. By analogy, no worries yet on this account with Cerazette® either—or with the IUS (below) whose amenorrhoeic action is anyway primarily at the end-organ level, the endometrium.

Contraindications

Absolute contraindications for DMPA

- Past *severe arterial* diseases, or current very high risk thereof (because of the above evidence about low oestrogen levels coupled with reports of lowered HDL cholesterol).
- Current osteopenia or severe risk factor(s) for osteoporosis, including chronic corticosteroid treatment (>5mg per day).
- Any serious adverse effect of COCs not certainly related solely to the oestrogen (e.g. liver adenoma or cancer, though WHOMEC classifies these as WHO 3).
- Recent breast cancer not yet clearly in remission (see below).
- Acute porphyria, even if latent, no history of actual attack (progestogens as well as oestrogens are believed capable of precipitating these and the injection is not 'removable').
- Undiagnosed genital tract bleeding.
- Actual or possible pregnancy.
- Hypersensitivity to any component.

Relative contraindications for DMPA (WHO 2 unless otherwise stated)

- According to degree, except as above arterial disease risk is WHO 3 or 2.
- Short-term steroid treatment, recovered anorexia nervosa with normal menstrual cycling: see above, these are usually WHO 3.
  - <18 or
  - >45 years of age
  are WHO 2 with respect to the bones (see above).
- Active liver disease with abnormal liver function tests—caution required (WHO 3)—but WHO 2 with normal biochemistry.
- Recent trophoblastic disease is WHO 3 (UKMEC) until hCG is undetectable in blood as well as urine, then WHO 1.
- DMPA is usable in all non-acute porphyrias (WHO 2).
- Sex steroid-dependent cancer, including breast cancer, in complete remission is WHO 3 (after 5yrs according to WHOMEC). However, a POP or LNG-IUS would be preferable (lower dose, more reversible).
- Unacceptability of menstrual irregularities, especially cultural/religious taboos whether associated with bleeding or amenorrhoea.
- Obesity, although further weight gain is not inevitable (see below).
- Past severe endogenous depression.
- Planning a pregnancy in the near future (see below).

Counselling and ongoing supervision

Four practical points must always be made to prospective users:
- The effects, whether wanted (contraceptive) or unwanted, are *not reversible for the duration of the injection*: this fact is unique among current contraceptives.
- After the last dose, *conception is commonly delayed* with a median delay of 9 months, which is of course only 6 months after cessation of the method, but in some individuals it could be well over 1yr.
- Weight gain is probable due to increased appetite, so it is useful (and can really work) to advise a pre-emptive plan to start taking extra exercise as well as watching diet.
- Irregular, sometimes prolonged *bleeding may be a problem*, but the outlook is good as usually followed after a few months by *amenorrhoea* which (it should be explained) is not a problem.

Follow-up

Apart from ensuring the injections take place at the correct intervals, follow-up is primarily advisory and supportive.
- Prolonged or too frequent bleeding is managed as already described.
- BP is normally checked initially but there is absolutely no need for it to be taken before each dose, as studies fail to show any hypertensive effect. An annual check is reasonable as well-woman care.

Contraceptive implants

Introduction

Implants contain a progestogen in a slow-release carrier, made either of dimethylsiloxane (as in Jadelle™ not available in UK) with two implants or of ethylene vinyl acetate (EVA) as Implanon®, a single rod (Fig. 25.1).

They are excellent examples of long-acting reversible contraceptive (LARCs) with the ideal 'forgettable' default state yet rapid reversibility.

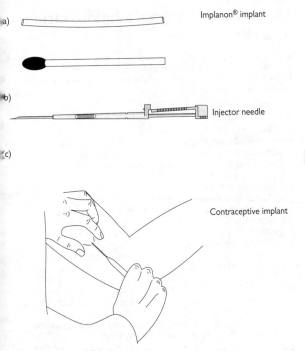

a)   Implanon® implant

b)   Injector needle

(c)   Contraceptive implant

Fig. 25.1 Implanon® contraceptive implant.

Mechanism of action, administration and effectiveness

- Implanon works primarily by ovulation inhibition, supplemented mainly by the usual sperm-blocking mucus effect of progestogen.
- It is a single 40mm rod, just 2mm in diameter, containing 68mg of etonogestrel—the chief active metabolite of desogestrel—and so has much in common with Cerazette®. This is dispersed in an EVA matrix and covered by a 0.06mm rate-limiting EVA membrane.

Clinically

- It is inserted subdermally over the biceps medially in the upper arm, with local anaesthesia, from a dedicated sterile preloaded applicator by a simple injection/withdrawal technique—aided by the blunt bevel of its cleverly shaped wide-bore needle.
- It is inserted *anterior* to the groove between the triceps and biceps, well away from the neurovascular bundle. After an initial phase of several weeks giving higher blood levels, Implanon® delivers almost constant low daily levels of the hormone, for a recommended duration of use of 3yrs.
- *Though this implant is much easier than Norplant® to insert or remove, specific (model arm plus live) training is essential and cannot be obtained from any book.* In the UK, the best training is obtainable through the FFP&RHC.
- Implanon® had the unique distinction of a zero failure rate in the premarketing trials, though the 'perfect use' (i.e. typical use) failure rate is now estimated as 5 in 10 000.
- Nearly all 'failures' that have been reported had had the insertion in a conception cycle or were failures to insert.

Effect of body mass

Serum levels tend to be lower in heavier women, but given the high margin of efficacy subsequently, failures have not been attributed to BMI.

Clinically

- This finding should *not* detract in the slightest from offering Implanon to overweight women for whom the COC (or Evra®) has a high VTE risk.
- *Earlier replacement?* The SPC says 'consider' this in the third year of use by 'heavier' women. This author would only discuss this possibility in a young fertile woman with a BMI well over 100kg if she began to cycle regularly in the third year (suggesting reliance only on the mucus effect).

Enzyme inducer drug (EID) treatment

- The SPC states that hepatic enzyme inducers may lower the blood levels of etonogestrel.
- Therefore, women on *short-term treatment* with any of these drugs are advised to use a barrier method in addition and (because reversal of enzyme induction always takes time) for 28 days thereafter.
- During *long-term EID treatment*, Organon has only one recommendation, to transfer to a non-hormonal method with removal of the Implanon®. However, given that Implanon® blood levels are ordinarily considerably higher in the first 18 months, another option to be considered—on a ☞ 'named patient' basis (📖 p. 431)—is early replacement, at 12–18 months. Another possibility, and probably more effective as well as cheaper for long-term users, is switching to either DMPA or the LNG-IUS: enzyme-inducer drug users do very well with either of these.

Reversibility and removal problems

Reversal is normally simple, with almost immediate effect:
- Under local anaesthetic, digital pressure on the proximal end of the Implanon® and a 2mm incision over the distal end leads to delivery of that end of the rod, removal being completed by grasping it with mosquito forceps.
- Again (see above), removal training is crucial, using the 'model arm' and live under supervision.

Removal problems, including discomfort, can be minimized by goo training, in both the insertion and removal techniques.

Difficult removals correlate with initially too-deep insertion. Bewar particularly of the thin or very muscular woman with very little subcuta neous tissue. Insertion can easily permit a segment of the rod to ente the (biceps) muscle, with deep migration ensuing.
- Specialized ultrasound techniques are required to localize 'lost' Implanons®, and removal may need to be under ultrasound control.

Indications

Being an anovulant, special indications include past ectopic pregnancy an
as a possibility for menstrual disorders, though the outcome is not reliab
beneficial (because of irregular bleeding, see below)

Advantages

- It provides efficacy and convenience: if the bleeding pattern suits, it is a 'forgettable' contraceptive.
- Long action with one treatment (3yrs); high continuation rates.
- Absence of the initial peak dose given orally to the liver.
- Blood levels are low and steady, rather than fluctuating (as with the POP) or initially too high (as with injectables); this with previous bullet minimizes metabolic changes.
- Oestrogen-free, therefore definitely usable if history of VTE (WHO 2).
- Median systolic and diastolic BP were unchanged in trials for up to 4yrs.
- The implant is rapidly reversible: after removal, serum etonogestrel levels were undetectable within 1 week. From the contraceptive point of view, return of fertility must be assumed to be almost immediate during the first week.

Disadvantages and contraindications

Contraindications are very similar to Cerazette® since, like it but unlike DMPA, Implanon® is an anovulant yet immediately reversible (and they contain essentially the same progestogen).

Local adverse effects occur, namely:
- infection of the site.
- expulsion.
- migration and difficult removal (see above) and
- scarring.

Absolute contraindications (WHO 4) for Implanon®
- Any serious adverse effect of COCs not certainly related solely to the oestrogen (e.g. liver adenoma or cancer: WHOMEC is more permissive, WHO 3).
- Recent breast cancer not yet clearly in remission (see below).
- Acute porphyria with history of actual attack precipitated by hormones, otherwise WHO 3.
- Known or suspected pregnancy.
- Undiagnosed genital tract bleeding.
- Hypersensitivity to any component.

The manufacturer adds 'severe hepatic disease', which WHOMEC classifies as WHO 3, and 'active venous thromboembolic disorder', which presumably means a current episode, which is WHO 3 according to WHOMEC. There is no evidence that Implanon® (like other progestogen-only methods) would increase VTE risk.

Relative contraindications (WHO 3)
- Acute porphyria, latent, with no previous attack (plus forewarning/monitoring); Implanon is also usable in all the non-acute porphyrias.
- Current severe liver disorder with persistent biochemical change.
- Recent trophoblastic disease until hCG is undetectable in blood as well as urine, then WHO 1.
- Sex steroid-dependent cancer, including breast cancer, in complete remission (WHO advises 5yrs). In all cases agreement of the relevant hospital consultant should be obtained and the woman's autonomy respected: record that she understands it is unknown whether progestogen alone in Implanon alters the recurrence risk.
- Enzyme inducers—discussed above. (But using another method such as an IUD or IUS would be preferable.)
- Past symptomatic functional ovarian cysts—*might* recur using Implanon especially in the third year

Relative contraindications (WHO 2)
- Past VTE or severe risk factors for VTE; clinically, in fact, this is often an indication, see above.
- Risk factors for arterial disease; more than one risk factor can be present.
- Current liver disorder (now) with normal biochemistry.

- Most other chronic severe systemic diseases.
- Unacceptability of irregular menstrual bleeding: which remains a problem with all progestogen-only methods, certainly including Implanon.

Timing of Implanon insertion

- In the woman's natural cycle, day 1–5 is usual timing; if any later than day 5 (assuming no sexual exposure up to that day) recommend additional contraception for 7 days.
- If a woman is on COC or POP/Cerazette or DMPA, the implant can normally be inserted any time, with no added precautions.
- *Clinical implications*: insertions only in the tiny natural-cycle window are a logistic and conception risk nightmare! So a useful practical tip is actively to recommend use of an anovulant method (i.e. one of those in last bullet) at counselling, for use until the Implanon insertion.
- Following delivery (not breastfeeding) or second-trimester abortion, insertion on about day 21 is recommended, or if later with additional contraception for 7 days. If later and still amenorrhoeic, pregnancy risk should be excluded (📖 p. 430–1).
- If breastfeeding, insert day 21–28 (UKMEC), with no need for added contraception for 7 days.
- Following first-trimester abortion, immediate insertion is best:
  - on the day of surgically induced abortion or second part of a medical abortion, or
  - up to 7 days later;
  - if >7 days later, an added method such as condoms is recommended for 7 days.

Counselling and ongoing supervision

- Explain the likely changes to the bleeding pattern and the possibility of 'hormonal' side-effects (see below). This discussion should as always be backed by a good leaflet, such as the FPA one, and well documented.
- No treatment-specific follow-up is necessary (including no need for BP checks). The SPC recommends one follow-up visit at 3 months.

Bleeding problems

In the pre-marketing RCT comparing Implanon® with the old 6-implant Norplant®, although amenorrhoea was significantly more common,
- the combined rates for the more annoying 'frequent bleeding and spotting' and 'prolonged bleeding and spotting' were very similar.

Clinical Management

After eliminating unrelated causes for the bleeding (📖 p. 329):
- ☞ The best short-term treatment is cyclical oestrogen therapy, here usually using Mercilon®, as explained for DMPA (📖 p. 364). The plan should be explained to the woman, who should also understand that it is not certain to work. Courses may be repeated if an acceptable bleeding pattern does not follow. Or:
- ☞ An alternative that was effective, though only short-term in a pilot study, is doxycycline 100mg bd for 5 days. The mechanism is believed to be an effect on endometrial enzymes and is probably independent of treating any Chlamydial endometritis. But one should test for Chlamydia first, as usual with irregular bleeding.
- ☞ Some clinicians report success from use of an added Cerazette® tablet daily for a few weeks at a time.

Minor side-effects

Reported in frequency order these were:
- acne (but this might also improve!)
- headache
- abdominal pain
- breast pain
- 'dizziness'
- mood changes (depression, emotional lability)
- libido decrease
- hair loss

Weight gain

In the above RCT, the mean body weight increase over 2yrs was 2.6% with Implanon® and 2.9% with Norplant®, while, in a parallel study, similar users of an IUD showed weight increases of 2.4% in the same time scale. Weight seems to be less of a problem than with DMPA, though some individuals do find their weight gain unacceptable.

Bone mineral density

Since Implanon® suppresses ovulation and does not supply any oestrogen the same questions as with DMPA arise over possible hypo-oestrogenism. However, it appears that, like Cerazette® and other POPs, the suppression of FSH levels with Implanon® is less complete, allowing adequate follicular phase oestrogen levels (ie usually not as low as the levels in DMPA users).

In a non-randomized comparative study, no bone density changes or differences were detected in either 44 Implanon® users or 29 users of copper IUDs over 2 years, which is reassuring.

Intra-uterine contraception

Introduction

Intra-uterine contraceptives are currently of two distinct types:

- copper intra-uterine devices, abbreviated as IUDs, in which the copper ion (the actual contraceptive) is released from a band or wire on a plastic carrier;
- levonorgestrel-releasing intra-uterine system which releases that progestogen. It will be abbreviated below as either LNG-IUS or just IUS.

Copper-bearing devices

Advantages of and indications for copper IUDs

- Safe: mortality 1:500 000.
- Effective:
  - immediately
  - postcoitally (but not true of the LNG-IUS)
  - like sterilization if one of the many clones of the T-Safe Cu 380A® is used (see below).
- No link with coitus.
- No tablets to remember.
- Continuation rates high and duration of use can exceed 10yrs.
- Reversible and there is evidence that this is true even when IUDs have been removed for one of the recognized complications.

Mechanism of action

Appropriate studies indicate that copper IUDs operate
- primarily by preventing fertilization, the copper ion being toxic to sperm. Their effectiveness when put in postcoitally shows that they
- can also act to block implantation.

However, when IUDs are *in situ* long term, this seems to be a rarely needed 2° or back-up mechanism.

Clinical implication
- Use another method additionally from 7 days before planned device removal, or if this has not been the case.
- postpone removal till the next menses.

If a device *must* be removed earlier, hormonal postcoital contraception may be indicated.

Choice of devices and effectiveness

In the UK, the 'gold standard' among IUDs for a parous woman without menstrual problems is any **banded copper IUD** (Fig. 26.1). Available are:
- **T-Safe Cu 380A**® or new variants with their copper bands sunk into the arms of the plastic frame, which are branded as **TT 380 'Slimline'**® or **T-Safe Cu 380A QL 'Quick Load'**®: available, respectively, from Durbin or FP Sales; see MIMS. The latter both have a simpler loading system than the fiddly plastic 'hat' of the older T-Safe Cu 380A®.

Important influence of age on effectiveness

Copper IUDs are much more effective in the older woman, largely because of declining fertility. Over the age of 30 there is also a reduction in rates of expulsion and of PID, the latter of which is not believed to be the result of the older uterus resisting infection but because the older woman is generally less exposed to risk of infection (whether through her own lifestyle or that of her only partner).

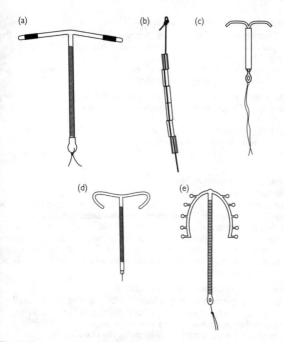

Fig. 26.1 Illustration of some current IUDs in the UK (please note: devices are not drawn to scale). (a) TT 380 Slimline®, (b) GyneFix®, (c) Mirena® (LNG-IUS), (d) Flexi-T 300®, (e) Multiload 375®.

Crown copyright material is reproduced with the permission of the Controller of HMSO.

Advantages of any of the banded IUDs

- Efficacy in one RCT was greater than the all-wire **Nova T 380®**, but the main advantage lies in the infrequency of re-insertions. Research in the past 50yrs has clearly shown that
    - most IUD complications can be insertion related and also
    - reduce in frequency with duration of use.

IUD Slogan 1: *'Insertion can be a factor in the causation of almost every category of IUD problems … therefore, why ever use a 5yr device when a 10yr one will fit?'*

- It is licensed for 10yrs and the data support effectiveness till **12yrs** (even when fitted below age 40, see below).
- It usually passes through the cervical canal surprisingly easily, in all parities.

What if the woman is nulliparous?

NB: Nulliparity *per se* is not WHO 4 for this method! In a mutually monogamous relationship especially above age 35 it should be seen as only WHO 2 for the IUD method. Available since mid-2007, and now the first choice for nulliparae, is the Mini TT 380® (Durbin), with reduced dimensions but the same amount of copper. Its insertion tube is no thinner yet it usually passes readily through the cervix. Otherwise for a comfortable and satisfactory fitting one of the small wire-bearing IUDs may be better (see options below).

When to use other IUDs, e.g. Nova T 380®?

- *Emergency contraception (EC)* **Nova T 380®** might be appropriate for a nulliparous woman *using it for EC* and planning to have the device removed once established on a new method (such as say DMPA). Another good EC option for nulliparae is **the Flexi-T 300®** which is exceptionally small and has an easy push-in fitting technique with no separate plunger. But it has been reported to have a highish expulsion rate.
- *For long-term use*, both **Nova T 380®** and the **UT 380 Short®** (Nova T style but on a shorter stem, from Durbin) are less ideal and should usually be reserved for when the T-Safe Cu 380A® or Mini TT 380® cannot be fitted, for some reason. The latter could be an unusually tight cervix or acute flexion of the uterus, rare in parous women but not uncommon in nulliparae.
- There is now also available the **Flexi-TT 380™**, on a slightly larger frame and with bands on its side arms but otherwise shaped as the Flexi-T 300®.
- The **Multiload IUDs®**, even the 375 thicker wire version, were (again) significantly less effective than the T-Safe Cu 380A® in WHO studies, *with no evidence of the reputed better expulsion rate.*

When to use the frameless banded GyneFix™?

- This unique frameless device features a knot that is embedded by its special inserter system in the fundal myometrium.
- Below the knot, its polypropylene thread bears six copper bands and locates them within the uterine cavity.

● Being frameless makes it less likely to cause uterine pain, and when correctly inserted it appears to rival the efficacy of the T-Safe Cu 380A®. Indications include:
  • Distorted cavity on ultrasound scan (if IUD useable at all), or
  • A small uterine cavity sounding <6cm—with no minimum. Rival and probably more available options down to minimum 5cm are the **UT 380™ Short or the (wire) Flexi-T 300®**.
  • Previous history of expulsion or removal of a framed device that was accompanied by excessive cramping, within hours or days of insertion.

Main problems and disadvantages of copper IUDs

The main medical problems are listed in the box below. This is actually a remarkably short list as compared with hormonal methods.

1. Intra-uterine pregnancy, hence its risk including miscarriage.
2. Extra-uterine pregnancy, prevented less well than intra-uterine, though absolute risk actually reduced in population terms.
3. Expulsion, hence the risks of pregnancy/miscarriage.
4. Perforation
   • risks to bowel/bladder
   • risks of pregnancy, again.
5. Pelvic infection—as with (2), the IUD is *not* causative.
6. Malpositioning (which predisposes to (1), (3) and (7)).
7. Pain.
8. Bleeding
   • increased amount
   • increased duration.

Note, clinically that

IUD Slogan 2: *Pain and bleeding in IUD users signify a potentially dangerous condition—until proved otherwise.* Meaning that: all of the first six problems need to be excluded as diagnoses before pain and bleeding are ascribed simply to being side-effects of this method.

In situ conception

If the woman wishes to go on to full-term pregnancy, after a pelvic ultrasound scan demonstrates an intra-uterine pregnancy, *the device should normally be removed.*

- spontaneous abortion was 55%, dropping to 20% if the device was removed.

Other clinical points

- If the woman is going to have a termination of her pregnancy, her IUD (or IUS) can be removed at the planned surgery; but it is safest to remove it before any medical abortion.
- If the threads are already missing when she is seen and other causes are excluded, aided by an ultrasound scan (see below), *the pregnancy is at increased risk,* of:
  - second-trimester abortion (which could be infected), and
  - antepartum haemorrhage, and
  - premature labour.
- If the woman goes on to full term, it is essential to identify clearly the device in the products of conception. If it is not found, a postpartum X-ray should be arranged in case the device is embedded or malpositioned, or has perforated.

There have been many medico-legal cases when this was not done, leading either to:
  - problems from an undiagnosed perforation or
  - unnecessary tests and treatments for 'infertility' when a much earlier malpositioned device with no visible threads had been left *in situ.*
- There is no evidence of associated **teratogenicity** with conception during or immediately after use of copper devices.

IUDs with 'lost threads'

IUD Slogan 3: The woman with 'lost threads' is already pregnant until proven otherwise—(moreover even then she is probably unprotected and at risk of becoming pregnant).

'Lost threads'—six possible causes

Pregnant	Not pregnant
Unrecognized expulsion + pregnancy	Unrecognized expulsion + not yet pregnant
Perforation + pregnancy	Perforation + not yet pregnant
Device in situ + pregnancy	Device in situ + malpositioned or threads short (in uterus, if not found in cervical canal)

Diagnosis and management may involve

- First, ascertaining if the threads are, in fact, present: they may perhaps be short and drawn up into the canal.
- Pregnancy testing.

- Imaging by ultrasound, sometimes also X-ray.
- Use of special extractors and forceps under local anaesthetic.
- Operative laparoscopy under general anaesthaetic.

The later stages of this progression should be after referral to a specialist.

More about perforation

This has a general estimated risk for all IUDs of ~1 per 1000 insertions, but the exact rate (like for expulsion) depends much less on the IUD design than on the skill of the clinician. Perforated devices should now almost always be removable at laparoscopy.

Pelvic inflammatory disease (PID) and IUDs—what is the truth?

IUD Slogan 4: *IUDs, intrinsically, cannot be the cause of the PID that occurs in IUD users* … Otherwise in China (with a vanishingly low incidence of PID at the time) there would have been at least one reported case among the 4301 IUD insertions, in the WHO database presented in Figure 26.2.

- The greatest risk is in the first 20 days, most probably caused by pre-existing carriage of STIs.
- Risk thereafter, as with preinsertion, relates to the background STI risk.

Therefore, the evidence-based policy should be that:

- Elective IUD insertions and reinsertions should always occur through a cervix that has been established to be pathogen-free, so hopefully eliminating the postinsertion infections in Fig. 26.2.

Clinical implications for IUD insertion arrangements

- Prospective IUD users should as always be verbally screened, meaning a good sexual history (Chapter 1, 📖 p. 262). They need to know that they will, at least, need to use condoms too if the method is judged WHO 3 because of high STI risk, or even use another method altogether (WHO 4).
- 'When did you last have sex with someone different?' means a rethink about the IUD method if that was within the past 3 months; also, and this is the thorny one, we all tend to leave out:
- 'Do you ever wonder if your partner has or is likely to have another sexual relationship?' (Always said or reworded with the utmost tact).
- In populations with high prevalence of *Chlamydia trachomatis* (say >5% incidence—and NB it is around twice that in most recent UK surveys of the under 25s), this should be backed by modern DNA-based (LCR or PCR) prescreening. This would be as important for reinsertions as for initial IUD insertions.
- Recent exposure history or evidence of a purulent discharge from the cervix indicates referral for more detailed investigation at a Genitourinary Medicine (GUM) clinic.
- If Chlamydia is detected, the woman should be referred to a GUM clinic:
  - investigated for linked pathogens,
  - necessary treatment and contact tracing arranged, and
  - the IUD insertion postponed.

In EC cases: screen but treat anyway before the result is available (e.g. with azithromycin 1g stat)

- The cervix should be cleansed very thoroughly (primarily physically, by swabbing) before any device is inserted, with minimum trauma following the manufacturer's instructions.
- In addition to the routine 6-week follow-up visit, a first postinsertion visit might be appropriate at 1–2 weeks, designed to identify any women with postinsertion infection (during the crucial 20 days of Fig. 26.2).
- As a minimum, the woman should be given clear details of the relevant symptoms of PID, and instructed as routine to telephone the practice nurse ~1 week postinsertion.

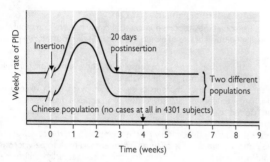

Fig. 26.2 WHO study of 22 908 IUD insertions (4301 in China) in Europe, Africa, Asia and the Americas. Note that the weekly rate of pelvic inflammatory disease (PID) returns to the preinsertion background rate for the population studied This figure also appears in John Guillebaud. *Contraception Today*. London: Martin Dunitz, 2004, 📖 p. 27.

Actinomyces-like organisms (ALOs)

These are sometimes reported in cervical smears, more commonly with increasing duration of use of either IUDs or IUSs. If reported:

A

First, call the woman for an extra consultation and examination, particularly bimanually. If all is normal , see below, but:

- If there are relevant symptoms or signs (pain, dyspareunia, excessive discharge, tenderness, any suggestion of an adnexal mass) then an ultrasound scan should then be arranged, with a low threshold for gynaecological referral.
- After preliminary discussion with the microbiologist, the device should be removed and sent for culture. Treatment will have to be vigorous, usually prolonged, if frank pelvic actinomycosis is actually confirmed— it is a potentially life-threatening and fertility-destroying condition, although very rare.

Second part of protocol on detection of ALOs

When there are no positive clinical findings, in consultation with the woman the clinician may decide between **EITHER**:

B

- Simple removal with or without reinsertion, and without antibiotic treatment.
- Advise the woman, along with written reference material, about the relevant symptoms which should make her seek a doctor urgently and tell them that she recently had an IUD or IUS plus ALOs.
- Repeat a cervical smear after 3 months (it will nearly always be negative) with a re-check bimanual examination. Both smear-taking and IUD follow-up then revert to normal arrangements.

OR

C

- Leave the IUD or IUS alone after the initial thorough and fully reassuring examination, preferably backed by a negative pelvic ultrasound scan.
- Advise the woman, along with written material, about the relevant symptoms which should make her seek a doctor urgently and tell them that she has been followed-up with an IUD or IUS plus ALOs.
- Arrange meticulous follow-up, initially at 6 months, including a check for symptoms and bimanual examination

✎ Given the data that device removal usually clears the ALO finding, even though long-term use is normally best, there is much to be said for following plan A+B rather than A+C above.

In either case, keep a good quality record of the consultation.

Is ectopic pregnancy caused by copper IUDs?

- Ectopic pregnancies are actually reduced in number because very few sperm get through the copper-containing uterine fluids to reach an egg, so very few implantations can occur in any damaged tube. However, there are even fewer implantations in the uterus. Thus, in the ratio of ectopic/intra-uterine pregnancies, the denominator is even lower than the numerator, allowing the ratio to increase, even though both types of pregnancy are actually reduced in frequency.
- A past history is a WHO 3 relative contraindication to the IUD in nulliparae since there are even better options which are anovulants, e.g. COC, Cerazette®, DMPA. The LNG-IUS is also relatively contraindicated, though only WHO 2. See ⊞ p. 402.

IUD Slogan 5: Any IUD user with pain and a late or unusually light period or irregular bleeding has an ectopic pregnancy until proved otherwise.

Pain and bleeding

Copper devices do increase

- The *duration* of bleeding by a mean of 1–2 days, and also
- The measured *volume* of bleeding by about one-third.

However if her periods are initially light and of short duration, any addition may be hardly noticeable by the woman.

Bleeding problems usually settle with time. If they do not, it may be necessary to change the method of contraception, perhaps to the LNG-IUS (see below).

Duration of use

IUD Slogan 6: Any copper device (even a copper-wire-only type) that has been fitted above the age of 40 may be used for the rest of reproductive life. It never needs replacement, even though it is not licensed for that long. For duration of use of the LNG-IUS in various situations, see below.

Cancer risk?

There is no increased cancer risk.

The levonorgestrel-releasing intra-uterine system (LNG-IUS, or Mirena®)

(Schering Health Care)

The unique LNG-IUS is shown in Fig. 26.3.

Method of action and effectiveness

Main features of the **LNG-IUS**

- It releases ~20 micrograms per 24h of LNG from its polydimethylsiloxane reservoir, through a rate-limiting membrane, for its licensed 5yrs (and longer).
- Its main contraceptive effects are local, through changes to the cervical mucus and uterotubal fluid which impair sperm migration, backed by endometrial changes impeding implantation.
- Its cumulative failure rate to 7yrs was very low, 1.1 per 100 women in the large Sivin study, and even less to 5yrs in the 1994 European multicentre trial.
- Its efficacy is not detectably impaired by enzyme-inducing drugs.
- The systemic blood levels of LNG are under half of the mean levels in users of the LNG POP (for users this can be explained as 'like taking 3 old-type POPs per week') and so though ovarian function is altered in some women, especially in the first year, 85% show the ultrasound changes of normal ovulation at 1yr.
- The amount of LNG in the blood is still enough to give unwanted hormone-type side-effects in some women; otherwise irregular light bleeding is the main problem.
- Even if they become amenorrhoeic—as many do, primarily through a local end-organ effect—in those who do not ovulate (as well as the majority who do), sufficient oestrogen is produced for bone health.
- Return of fertility after removal is rapid and appears to be complete.

Different though it is to other intrauterine methods, all the 6 IUD 'slogans given above do also apply to the LNG-IUS (with one small age change to >45 for slogan 6 (📖 p. 403)).

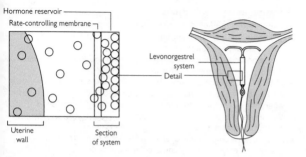

Fig. 26.3 The levonorgestrel-releasing intra-uterine system (LNG-IUS)
Reproduced from *The Pill* part of the Facts series. 6th edition. By permission of Oxford University Press.

Advantages and indications
The user of this method can expect the following advantages
- A dramatic reduction in amount and, *after the first few months* (discussed below), duration of blood loss.
- Dysmenorrhoea is improved in most women and (for unexplained reasons) the symptoms of PMS in some.
- The LNG-IUS is the *contraceptive* method of choice for most women with menorrhagia or who are prone to iron-deficiency anaemia. Even when there is no need for contraception it should still be seen in primary care as the first-line treatment for excessively heavy menses without major cavity distortion, and is fully licensed as such.
- HRT: by providing progestogenic protection of the uterus during oestrogen replacement by any chosen route, it uniquely, before final ovarian failure, offers 'forgettable, contraceptive, no-period and no PMS-type HRT'. For this increasingly popular indication, the LNG-IUS is currently licensed for 4yrs before it must be replaced.
- Epilepsy: in a small series at the MPC this was a very successful method for this condition, even in women on enzyme inducer treatment.
- The LNG-IUS is, in short, a highly convenient and 'forgettable' contraceptive—with added gynaecological value.

What about infection/ectopic pregnancy risk and risk to future fertility?
- LNG-IUS may actually reduce the frequency of clinical PID, perhaps through the progestogenic effect on cervical mucus, particularly in the youngest age groups who are most at risk.
- *However,* the risk is certainly not eliminated and (outside of mutual monogamy) condom use should still be advocated.
- Future fertility is most unlikely to be adversely affected.
- *Reduction in ectopic risk*—this can be attributed to its greater efficacy by the sperm-blocking mechanism that reduces the risk of pregnancy in any site. However ectopics still rarely occur and, with a past history of an ectopic pregnancy, an anovulant method would be *even better*.

Problems and disadvantages of the LNG-IUS
As with any IUD:
- *Expulsion* can occur and there is the usual small risk of
- *Perforation*, minimized by its 'withdrawal' as opposed to 'plunger' technique of insertion.
- A more important problem is the high incidence in the first postinsertion months of *uterine bleeding* which, although small in quantity, may be very frequent or continuous and can cause considerable inconvenience. In later months:
- *Amenorrhoea* is common but should be explained being an advantage!

Women can accept the early weeks of light bleeding, even if very frequent, as a worthwhile price to pay for all the other advantages of the method: provided they are well informed in advance of LNG-IUS fitting.
- Women should also be forewarned that although this method is mainly local in its action it is not exclusively so. Therefore, there is a small incidence of *'hormonal' side-effects* such as bloatedness, acne and

depression. These do usually improve, often within 2 months, in parallel with the known decline in the higher initial LNG blood levels.

• Functional ovarian cysts are also more common, although they are usually asymptomatic. If pain results, they should be investigated/monitored but will usually resolve spontaneously.

Contraindications

Many of the contraindications of this method are shared with copper IUDs (see below). The additional few that are unique to LNG-IUS, due to the actions of its LNG hormone, are discussed in the box below. The manufacturer tends to be more cautious in calling them all WHO 4.

Unique contraindications (mainly WHO 3) for LNG-IUS

• Current liver tumour or severe active hepatocellular disease (WHO 3).
• Current severe active arterial disease (WHO 2 according to WHOMEC).
• ☞ Current breast cancer. This is WHO 4 according to WHOMEC, with LNG-IUS usable on WHO 3 basis after 5yrs remission. In selected cases, this WHO 3 status might be agreed sooner, after consultation with the oncologist, given the risks and likelihood of pregnancy with other methods.
• Trophoblastic disease (any)—WHO 3 while blood hCG levels are high, as for other progestogen-only methods (UK advice), but no problem (WHO 1) after full recovery.
• Hypersensitivity to levonorgestrel or other constituent (WHO 4).

In addition, the LNG-IUS should not be used as a postcoital intra-uterine contraceptive (failures reported); using a hormone it appears not to act as quickly as the intra-uterine copper ion does.

Relative contraindications for copper IUDs also apply to the LNG-IUS method, but are usually less strong, except for bleeding and pain which indeed are positive indications (WHO 1).

Duration of use of the LNG-IUS in the older woman

The product is licensed for 5yrs.

• ☞ For contraception, effective use is evidence based but unlicensed for up to 7yrs. For a woman under age 35, because of her greater fertility, replacement after the usual 5yrs would be advisable. If fitted above that age it might be used for longer, even to 7 years, at a woman's fully empowered request, but always on a 'named-patient' basis (☐ p. 436).
  • NICE has stated that a woman who had her LNG-IUS inserted above the age of 45 with complete amenorrhoea may continue to use the same LNG-IUS 'until contraception is no longer needed'.
• As part of HRT, current practice for safe endometrial protection would be always to change at 4yrs.
• But if the LNG-IUS is not being and will not be used for either contraception or HRT, it could be left in situ for as long as it continues to work, in the control of heavy and/or painful uterine bleeding, and then removed after ovarian failure can be finally assured.

Main established contraindications to IUDs

NB these apply to the LNG-IUS as well, except where stated.

Absolute—but perhaps temporary—contraindications (WHO 4) for IUDs

- Suspicion of *pregnancy*.
- Undiagnosed *irregular genital tract bleeding*.
- *Significant infection*: postseptic abortion, current pelvic infection or STI, undiagnosed pelvic tenderness/deep dyspareunia or purulent cervical discharge.
- *Significant immunosuppression*, i.e. more profound than merely use of low-dose corticosteroids.
- Malignant or benign *trophoblastic disease, while hCG abnormal* (according to UKMEC; WHOMEC is less cautious. Both agree WHO 1 when hCG undetectable.)
- (LNG-IUS only) *Breast cancer*, becoming WHO 3 in remission (see 📖 p. 403) However, this might be an *indication* for copper IUD.

Absolute permanent contraindications (WHO 4) for IUDs

- Markedly *distorted uterine cavity*, or cavity sounding to *<5cm depth*. (But this is only WHO 2 for GyneFix).
- Known true *allergy to a constituent*.
- *Wilson's disease* (copper IUDs only).
- *Pulmonary hypertension*, because risk of fatal vasovagal reaction through cervical instrumentation.
- Previous *endocarditis*, or after *prosthetic valve replacement* (LNG-IUS can be WHO 3 for these, as it is believed the progestogen effect on mucus reduces risk of infection/endocarditis. But full antibiotic cover is required for insertion, see point 8 below).

Relative contraindications (WHO 2 unless otherwise stated) for IUDs

A longish list but in general meaning an IUD or the LNG-IUS is certainly usable with caution. Note again the differences specific to the LNG-IUS.

1. *Nulliparity and young age*, especially <20yrs. Though this is WHO 2 for fear of infection and the more serious implications should that happen (with no babies yet), this just means 'Broadly usable'. Both IUDs and IUSs are used successfully by many (carefully selected) women.
2. Lifestyle of self or partner(s) risking STIs. Combined with point 1, this equates to WHO 4, rarely 3 (but only with committed condom use).
3. Past *history of definite pelvic infection*.
4. Recent *exposure to high risk of a STI* (e.g. after rape—WHO 3). In emergency situations, such as for postcoital contraception, a copper IUD may be permissible (WHO 3) with full antibiotic cover (and after microbiological swabs are taken).
5. Known *HIV infection*. While controlled by drug therapy this is only WHO 2. LNG-IUS is better still because of reduced blood loss (added condom use routinely advised anyway).
6. Past *history of ectopic pregnancy* or other history suggesting high ectopic risk in a nullipara (WHO 3). T-Safe Cu 380A® or LNG-IUS are preferred IUDs: but regardless of parity it is even better to use an anovulant contraceptive.

7. *Suspected subfertility* already. WHO 2 for any cause, or WHO 3 if it relates to a tubal cause.

8. *Structural heart disease with risk of endocarditis.* but no history thereof (see above). WHO 3, signifying need for full antibiotic cover for IUD or IUS insertion as advised in the BNF. LNG-IUS probably better for these cases than a copper IUD, as believed to pose less ongoing infection risk due to the mucus effect.

9. *Any prosthesis which can be prejudiced by blood-borne infection*, e.g. hip replacement. IUDs are certainly usable, but termed WHO 2 to flag up preference for antibiotic cover for the insertion.

10. *Postpartum*, between 48h and 4 weeks (excess risk of perforation; WHO 3).

11. *Fibroids or congenital abnormality of uterus* with some but not marked distortion of the uterine cavity (see above). WHO 2 for framed IUDs or IUSs, WHO 1 for GyneFix®.

12. Severely *scarred/distorted uterus*, e.g. after myomectomy (WHO 3)

13. After *endometrial ablation/resection*—risk of IUD becoming stuck in shrunken and scarred cavity. LNG-IUS or GyneFix® usable in selected cases.

14. *Heavy periods*, with or without anaemia before insertion for any reason, including anticoagulation. This is an indication for the LNG-IUS (WHO 1).

15. *Dysmenorrhoea, any type.* LNG-IUS may well benefit this, provided the frame does not cause spasmodic pain.

16. *Endometriosis.* May be benefited by LNG-IUS (WHO 1), to help local symptoms in addition to systemic treatment.

17. *Diabetes.* WHO 2 for infection risk, but the IUD and LNG-IUS can be excellent choices.

18. *Penicillamine* treatment. 'Small print', unproven risk of causing copper IUD failure; LNG-IUS not affected.

19. *Previous perforation* of uterus This is WHO 2, almost WHO 1, at least for the small defect in the uterine fundus after a previous IUD perforation. Healing is so complete usually within 3 months, it is difficult even to locate the site of the previous event.

20. (LNG-IUS only) *Liver tumour or cancer* (WHO 3 because there is some systemic progestogen).

Note: if available and a copper IUD desired, GyneFix®, being frameless, would often be preferable for points 11–13.

The LNG-IUS is often best for 5, 8, 13–18.

Counselling, insertion and follow-up

Timing of insertions—all intra-uterine contraceptives
Generally:

- *In the normal cycle*, timing must avoid an already implanted pregnancy With copper IUDs (because they are such efficient postcoital methods), insertion can be at any time up to 5 days after the calculated day of ovulation, but not so with the LNG-IUS (see below).

- Postpartum insertions of IUDs or IUSs are usually at 6 weeks and acceptable from 4 weeks (beware increased risk of perforation). After 4 weeks if the woman is not fully breastfeeding, conception risk should be discussed (📖 p. 430) and additional contraception also advised for 7 days.
- Following first-trimester abortion (but only after preliminary counselling and full agreement by the woman), immediate insertion is best:
  - on the day of surgically induced abortion or second part of a medical abortion, if the uterus clearly empty—can check by on-the-spot ultrasound.

Additional points about insertion timing for the LNG-IUS

- In the normal cycle. Insertion for the IUS should be no later than day 7 of the normal cycle, since it does not operate as an effective postcoital contraceptive **and** because, in addition, any fetus might be harmed by conception in the first cycle (very high local LNG concentration).

Later insertion is also acceptable, but only if there has been believable abstinence beforehand and with continued contraception (e.g. condoms) postinsertion, for 7 days.

- If a woman is on COC or POP/Cerazette® or DMPA, the IUS can normally be inserted any time, with no added precautions. As with Implanon®, therefore (📖 p. 385), it is ideal to arrange that one of those methods is in use at the time of IUS-fitting.

Counselling and follow-up (for both IUDs and IUS)

After considering the contraindications, there should be an unhurried discussion with the woman of all the main practical points about this method, focusing on infection risk and the importance of reporting pain as a symptom at any time—and of telephoning if it occurred in the first 3 weeks postinsertion.

The only important routine follow-up visit is usually at 6 weeks after insertion. This is to:
- discuss with the woman any menstrual (or other) symptoms;
- check for (partial) expulsion;
- exclude infection, i.e. no relevant symptoms, tenderness or mass.

According to WHO, there need be no planned visits thereafter, relying on a fully understood 'open-house' policy. This is fine for copper IUDs, but extra visits in early months can sometimes be helpful for LNG-IUS users to maintain their motivation while their bleeding problems settle (see below).

Training for the actual insertion process

The Faculty of Family Planning (FFPRHC) training which leads to the Letter of Competence in Intrauterine Techniques is strongly recommended.

Good analgesia is crucial:

- Premedication with a prostaglandin inhibitor, e.g. mefenamic acid 500mg while in the waiting room, should be routine for all insertions.
- Local anaesthesia by intracervical injection should be taught and offered as a choice. It should almost always be used if the cervix has to be dilated or the uterine cavity explored.
- Moreover, there is a very unpredictable but sometimes bad pain which any woman (even a relaxed parous woman) may experience, caused by the application of the tenaculum at 12 o'clock on the cervix; and an initial 1mL dose of 1% lidocaine completely abolishes this.

As we have already noted, it is worth getting all aspects of insertion training right, since as we have already noted:

IUD Slogan 1: *Insertion can be a factor in the causation of almost every category of IUD problems.*

Moreover, the trainee's expertise must also be maintained long term thereafter, through regular practice.

Table 27.1 Emergency contraception: *choice of methods*

	LNG EC	Copper IUD
	LNG 1.5mg as stat dose	Immediate insertion, but sometimes better to delay (see text)
Normal timing after intercourse	Up to 72h but also usable up to 120h (see text)	Up to 5 days, or 5 days after earliest calculated day of ovulation
Efficacy (overall) within 72h	~99%	About 99.9%
Side-effects	Nausea 23% (15%) Vomiting 6% (1.4%)	Pain, bleeding, risk of infection

Reprinted with permission from Elsevier WHO. *Lancet* 1998; **352**: 428–33. WHO. *Lancet* 2002; **360**: 1803–10. (This study showed the lower rate of side effects in parentheses above.)

Levonorgestrel emergency contraception (LNG EC)

Mechanism of action

- *Given at or before ovulation* the method
  - interferes with follicle development, either inhibiting altogether or *delaying* ovulation.
- *Given later in a cycle* capable of inhibiting implantation, but this seems to be the less effective of its mechanisms—so the failure rate tends to be higher for sexual exposures late in the cycle.

Effectiveness and advantages

- Greater effectiveness: 99.6% when treatment began *within 24h of a single exposure*, compared with 98% for COEC.
- Reduced rates of the main side-effects of nausea and vomiting.
- In ordinary practice, there are virtually no contraindications to it.

The apparent effectiveness of LNG EC with treatment up to 72h after a single sexual exposure is ~99%, but this represents prevention of only 80% of the expected pregnancies: since most of those who present would not actually have conceived.

Enzyme inducer drug (EID) treatment

If the woman is taking one of these, hormonal EC is WHO 3. As usual, this category means it would be better to use an alternative, in this case:

- Insertion of a copper IUD (the more effective option), or
- if that is not acceptable, the dose should be doubled, i.e. two tablets totalling 3mg stat (unlicensed use).

The same applies if the woman is currently taking St John's Wort ('Nature's Prozac'), which is an enzyme inducer. But no increase in dose is needed when non-enzyme-inducing antibiotics are in use.

Warfarin users should have their INR checked 3–4 days after LNG EC, since it may alter significantly.

Contraindications

Absolute contraindications (WHO 4) to the hormone methods are essentially non-existent (WHOMEC)—those that may just be include:

- Current pregnancy.
- Proven severe allergy or intolerance to a constituent.
- Active acute porphyria, with a past attack precipitated by sex hormones.
- If the woman's own ethics preclude intervention postcoitally (or. more relevantly, postimplantation, see below).

Relative contraindications
- EID treatment, see above (WHO 3).
- Current breast cancer (WHO 3 due to uncertainty, but adverse effect unlikely with such short exposure).
- Trophoblastic disease with high hCG levels (WHO 2, as adverse effect unlikely and given the immediate risks of pregnancy).
- In breastfeeding, conception risk is of course usually very low so EC treatment would rarely be needed. If it is indicated (WHO 2), the infant could be bottle-fed for 24h, with expression of the breast milk.

Copper intrauterine devices (IUDs)

Insertion of a copper IUD—not the LNG-IUS—before implantation is extremely effective, through the toxicity of copper ions to sperm or by blocking implantation. This means, after consultation with the woman, that insertion may proceed *in good faith*, up to 5 days after:

• The first sexual exposure (regardless of cycle length); **or**
• The (earliest) calculated ovulation day. This entails:
   • calculate the *soonest likely* next menstrual start day
   • subtract 14 days for mean life of the corpus luteum and
   • add 5 days to allow for mean interval from fertilization to implantation.

Effectiveness

The copper IUD prevents conception in ~99.9% of women who present, or 98% of those who might be expected otherwise to conceive: even in cases of multiple exposure ever since the last menstrual period.

Indications for EC by copper IUD

In selected individuals (see the box below) IUD insertion may be ideal:

• When maximum efficacy is the woman's priority.
• When exposure occurred >72h earlier, or in cases of multiple exposure: insertion may be
   • up to 5 days after the earliest UPSI at any time in a cycle or
   • if there have been many UPSI acts, no later than 5 days after calculated ovulation.
• To be retained as their long-term method of contraception.
• In presence of contraindications to the hormonal method.
• If the woman is currently vomiting; or unexpectedly vomits her dose of LNG EC within 2h—in a case with particularly high pregnancy risk.

Clinically, given the sexual history, insertion in most cases should be:
• after microbiological cervical screening (at least for *Chlamydia trachomatis*) and also
• with prophylactic antibiotic cover, e.g. with azithromycin 1g stat, and
• with contact tracing to follow if STI test results later prove positive.

Counselling and management

- Preserve confidentiality.
- Evaluate the possibility of sexual assault or rape.
- Using a good leaflet, such as that of the FPA, as the basis for discussion, help the woman to make a fully informed and autonomous choice.
- This could be *either* of the two EC methods, *or* taking no action postcoitally.

Pharmacists should ensure privacy for the discussion and have a low threshold to refer all cases outside their specified remit (e.g. >72h since the earliest UPSI), to an appropriate clinical provider.

- Careful assessment of *menstrual/coital history* is essential.
- *Contraindications*. The mode of action may itself pose the only contraindication/problem for some individuals. Sometimes it may help to explain that there are circumstances when LNG EC's powerful prefertilization effects can remove concern about it needing to use the postfertilization mechanism (e.g. if the treatment is clearly going to be given well before ovulation in a given cycle—even though postcoitus).
- *Medical risks* should be discussed, at least in the leaflet, especially:
  - the *failure rate* (see above), reminding the woman that these figures relate to a single exposure. The failure rate is very close to nil for the IUD method;
  - *teratogenicity*: this is believed to be negligible;
  - *ectopic pregnancy*: if this occurs, the EC was not causative.

However:
  - a past history of ectopic pregnancy or pelvic infection remains a reason for specific forewarning with any of the methods,
  - **all** women should be warned to report back urgently if they get **pain**; and providers must 'think ectopic' whenever LNG EC or a copper IUD fails, or there is an odd bleeding pattern post-treatment.
- *Side-effects*: nausea occurs in 15%, vomiting in 1.4% of users. If the contraceptive dose is vomited within 2h, the woman may be given a further tablet with an anti-emetic: the best seems to be domperidone 10mg.
- *Contraception*, both
  - in the current cycle (in case the LNG EC method merely postpones ovulation), often condoms,
  and
  - long term should be discussed. The IUD option may cover both aspects (for a suitable long-term user). If the COC or injectable is chosen, it should normally be started as soon as the woman is convinced her next period is normal, usually on the first or second day, without the need for additional contraception thereafter.
- But 'Quick Start' of the COC is also an option in selected cases: meaning starting a COC immediately after the EC along with advice for 7 days of added condom use and hopefully 100% follow-up. The clinician must be confident that the benefits (especially to future compliance) outweigh the risks of EC failure. This is unlicensed, so should be on a 'named-patient' basis (📖 p. 436), with appropriate documented warnings.

Follow-up
- Women receiving LNG EC are rarely seen again routinely, but should be instructed to return:
  - if they experience pain or
  - their expected period is >7 days late, or lighter than usual.
- IUD acceptors return usually in 4–6 weeks for a routine check-up; or perhaps device removal, once established on what for them is a more appropriate long-term method.

Special indications for EC

These apply to coital exposure when the following have occurred:

- **Omission of anything more than two COC tablets** after the PFI, or of more than two pills in **the first 7 in the packet**.
- **Delay in taking a POP tablet for >3h**, outside of lactation, implying loss of the mucus effect, or of a Cerazette® tablet for >12h, followed by sexual exposure before mucus-based contraception was restored. The POP or Cerazette® is restarted immediately after the emergency regimen, 2 days added precautions are advised, and follow-up agreed.
- **If the POP user is breastfeeding**, EC would only be indicated if either the breastfeeding or the POP taking were unusually inadequate (⬚ p. 344).
- **Removal or expulsion of an IUD** before the time of implantation, if another IUD cannot be inserted, for some reason.
- **Further exposure in the same cycle**, e.g. due to failure of barrier contraception >1 day after a dose of EC has been taken. Additional courses of LNG EC are supported by the UKMEC, 'if clinically indicated', given reasonable precautions to avoid treating after implantation (repeated use thereafter will not induce an abortion).

This use is, again, outside the terms of the licence.

- **Use of LNG EC later than 72h after earliest UPSI**. This possibility has been tested, in the RCT by WHO (2002-ref ⬚ p. 411). The failure rate was low: only eight failures in 314 women treated between 72 and 120h (5 days) after the earliest act of UPSI. Though this was a small study and the confidence intervals were wide, this makes it sufficiently evidence based (though not yet licensed) for LNG EC to be offered to selected women in the 72–120h time period. They should be told of the limited evidence of efficacy, though it is 'likely to be better than doing nothing', and informed also that a copper IUD would definitely be more effective.
- **Overdue injections of DMPA with continuing sexual intercourse**. If it is later than day 91 (end of the 13th week): after a negative sensitive pregnancy test, LNG EC may be given along with the next injection **plus** advice to use condoms for 7 days. But after day 98 (14 weeks), the next injection is best postponed until there has been a total of 14 days of safe contraception or abstinence since the last exposure and a sensitive (< 25mIU/L) pregnancy test is negative—again with 7 days' added precautions and good follow-up.
- **Advanced provision of LNG EC**; UKMEC supports this in selected cases, to increase early use when required, e.g. to cover the risk of condom rupture or refusal of the partner to use when travelling abroad.

In all circumstances of use of EC, the women should be aware (as in the FPA leaflet), that

- the method might fail,
- it is not an abortifacient and
- it is given too soon to be able to harm a baby.

Sterilization

Introduction

Many individuals who say it is 'impossible' to accept continuing use of reversible contraceptives may just need updating to correct misinformation about the greater effectiveness and some added advantages of modern options they had not heard of (above all the LNG-IUS, but also the T-Safe 380 A® IUD and Implanon™).

Deferment or even avoidance of surgery is often ideal, through careful discussion and explanation of alternatives, particularly the long-acting reversible methods (LARCs).

Potential reversibility

Reported success of *reversal* procedures (male or female) depends enormously on patient selection, especially:

* how much damage was done at the initial procedure.
* the age of the woman in the new relationship.
* for vasectomy, time elapsed since surgery (poor results beyond 10yrs).

With competent microsurgery, as a rule of thumb, 80–90% tubal patency is usual.[1]

This surgery is not available everywhere and is usually expensive.

It is wise, therefore, to proceed with sterilization only when both partners can fully accept its permanence.

[1] Winston RM. Microsurgical tubocornual anastomosis for reversal of sterilisation. *Lancet* 1977; **1**: 284–285.

Possible long-term side-effects of female sterilization

- **The psychological sequelae** Considerable regret has been reported in 2% at 6 months and by 4% at 18 months, and postoperative psychiatric disturbance and dissatisfaction were largely associated with preoperative psychiatric disturbance. Higher rates of regret are reported when the sterilization is done at times that are not, except in rare special cases, now recommended: at termination of pregnancy or Caesarean section, or immediately postpartum.
- **Menstrual irregularity or menorrhagia** Sterilization, male or female, does not affect menstrual loss. However, if the method of contraception prior to the sterilization was COC, then the lighter regular withdrawal bleeds of the COC are replaced by normal menstruation. Therefore, counselling MUST include specific questioning about whether heavy bleeding or pain are or were problems during the woman's natural cycles, even if this relates to many years previously. Only with this information can the right decision be made, which could be to use the LNG-IUS instead of either party being sterilized.
- **Ovarian cancer** It appears in several studies that tubal sterilization may reduce the risk of ovarian cancer. This possible *beneficial side-effect* is difficult to explain, but may be a real effect.

Likelihood of regret following sterilization

A study in 1980 of women undergoing reversal of sterilization found

- 87% were under the age of 30. Marriages or intended long-term relationships started under age 25 in the UK now have a failure rate of >50%.
- 63% had been sterilized after delivery; and
- no less than 75% had been unhappy in their relationship.

It is of importance that any disharmony or pressurizing by the partner be identified. Easily missed, they are at least potentially more easily picked up by the referring clinician in primary care, as compared with the hospital gynaecologist or surgeon.

Decision making—mnemonic: 'LOVED REFERS'

L EAFLET—supplied by fpa in the UK or downloaded from www.rcog.org.uk.

O THER OPTIONS?—especially the LARCs such as the LNG-IUS, must be discussed. Also 'OPERATIONS', describe what they involve.

V ASECTOMY?—if LARC rejected, has this been considered?

E FFICACY—discuss (details above).

D ISHARMONY?—attempt to exclude problems in the couple's relationship by counselling and observing their body language.

R EVERSIBILITY—explain how difficult this might be, therefore the need to proceed as though it was irreversible. Also 'RISKS', of either procedure.

E CTOPIC—all women sterilized should be advised about the symptoms of this long-term risk.

F AMILY PLANNING—couple should avoid conception risk up to the date of the procedure. (A sensitive pregnancy test is now part of pre-operative routine.) The COC may be continued, since it does not pose an excess risk of thrombosis at laparoscopy.

E XAMINATION, AFTER GYNAE HISTORY—essential to ensure the right procedure done (e.g. may strongly indicate offering an LNG-IUS, or if fibroids are detected hysterectomy might be the preferred sterilizing procedure).

R EPLIES/RECORDS—i.e. answer the couple's questions and keep good records of the whole consultation.

S IGNATURE—applied, to standard Consent Form!

Comparison of methods

Vasectomy is very simple and medically safe under local anaesthesia. The method of choice is 'no scalpel vasectomy' (RCOG Guideline).

Sperm testing is usually done 12–16 weeks postsurgery, for two reasons, to:
- establish clearance of 'downstream' sperm and to
- exclude *early* failures of the procedure (incidence ~1%).

Clinically, men choosing vasectomy should be specifically advised
- in the short term about occasional large postoperative haematomas and
- longer term, about chronic postvasectomy scrotal pain. A surprisingly high incidence of this has been reported in some studies. Less than 1% of men seek medical help for this or report that it '. . . noticeably affects their quality of life'. It rarely seems to cause regret about having the vasectomy.

Despite concerns from timt to time, including about a link with testicular or prostate cancer, no long-term systemic risks have been established.

Tubal occlusion remains a more invasive procedure with risk of intra-abdominal injury even when performed under local anaesthesia. Confers immediate sterility (provided fertilization has not already occurred that cycle) while it may be several months before the semen is clear of sperm after the male operation.

More importantly, especially once she passes the age of 40, the woman is unlikely to wish for restoration of her fertility, even with any future new partner; and after her menopause Nature will dictate that she loses that option. Following vasectomy, however, if his partner should die or the relationship break down even beyond age 50, the man often finds a younger partner, with, accordingly, a much higher chance that as a new couple they will request a reversal procedure.

For more detail, the reader is referred to:
- The comprehensive RCOG National Guideline on male and female sterilization (containing all references alluded to above).
- The associated Summary document.

The exceptionally good patient information leaflet—all downloadable from: www.rcog.org.uk/index.asp? Page ID=699.

Special considerations

How can a provider be reasonably sure that a woman is not—or not about to be—pregnant?

WHO SPR advises that the provider can be reasonably certain that the woman is not pregnant if she has no symptoms nor signs of pregnancy and one or more of the following criteria apply:

- She has not had intercourse since last normal menses.
- She has been correctly and consistently using a reliable (sic) method of contraception.
- ➤ She is within the first 7 days after (onset of) normal menses.
- She is within 4 weeks postpartum for non-lactating women.
- She is within the first 7 days postabortion or miscarriage.
- She is fully or nearly fully breastfeeding, amenorrhoeic and <6 months postpartum.

In the UK, as appropriate, these criteria can be backed by a urine pregnancy test with sensitivity at least 25IU/L, best on a concentrated early morning sample.

Quick Start

Immediate starting of (usually) a pill method at first visit, late in the menstrual cycle or straight after EC. This may often be an entirely appropriate unlicensed use, but only when the above criteria have been applied so the provider is reasonably sure of a woman not being nor just about to be pregnant.

Secondary amenorrhoea, wants to (re-)start contraception

This is where the greatest difficulty arises, e.g.

- not breastfeeding and beyond 4 weeks postpartum, without reliable contraception to date, or
- a woman >2 weeks overdue her DMPA injection.

A pair of visits may often be required, since a prediagnosable pregnancy (unimplanted blastocyst) might be present at the first one.

First visit

Take history of early symptoms of pregnancy (increased micturition, nausea) and do a urine pregnancy test with sensitivity at least 25IU/L (only) if the history is suggestive. If this test is negative and there are no symptoms and **IF** more assurance is required before taking action (as for example before inserting a LNG-IUS):

- recommend her to abstain (preferable) or
- teach her to use a back-up method such as condoms with exceptional care or
- ☞ if neither of the above are appropriate, given that POPs have never been suspected of harming an early pregnancy, one of these may be prescribed.

UNTIL at least 14 days have elapsed since whenever was her last unprotected intercourse.

She should normally return at that time bringing an early morning urine sample. But if a pill method is planned, she may be given supplies in case her period comes on and she can start it at home as usual.

Second visit
- If she returns after menses, start any chosen method (including IUD or IUS) in the usual manner.
- If she returns still amenorrhoeic, do pregnancy test.

If now:
  - she has no symptoms of pregnancy plus
  - pregnancy test with sensitivity ≤25IU/L is negative and
  - the back-up method has reportedly been used well.

provide the (new) contraceptive method. If it is hormonal, advise usual back-up for 7 days or 2 days in the case of a POP.

Given that in 10–15% of cases a sensitive pregnancy test 14 days postcoitally can be falsely negative, arrange for a further follow-up in 2–4 weeks to confirm her non-pregnant state. Or at least instruct the woman to return if she develops symptoms which could be pregnancy—or fails to see her first withdrawal bleed on the COC.

Contraception at the climacteric

Maximum age for COC use

- *Smokers or others with arterial risk factors* should always discontinue the COC at age 35 (WHO 4). Pending more data, if they request a hormonal contraceptive they should use a POP or implant, but an IUD or IUS would be even better, or a vasectomy.

In selected healthy migraine-free, non-smokers, with modern pills and careful monitoring,

- the many gynaecological and other benefits of COCs are now felt to outweigh the small, though increasing, cardiovascular (and breast cancer) risk of a modern pill up to age 50–51, which is the mean age of the menopause.

Though there are usually much better contraceptive choices—consider especially an intra-uterine method—an appropriate COC (usually a 20 micrograms product) may therefore be used till then. For women with diminishing ovarian function but who need contraception as well, this is logical and preferable to HRT along with having to use some other contraceptive (though not advised beyond about age 50, see below).

Beyond 50 years of age, the age-related increased COC risks are usually unacceptable for all, given that fertility is now so low that simple, virtually risk-free contraceptives will suffice, e.g. spermicides, sponges or the POP.

Most forms of HRT are not contraceptive, but may be indicated combined with a simple contraceptive in symptomatic women when oestrogen is no longer being supplied by the COC. Of course, the IUS plus HRT combination is a winner here, since before final ovarian failure it safely supplies contraceptive HRT with endometrial protection plus, usually, highly acceptable amenorrhoea.

Diagnosing loss of fertility at the menopause

Although hormones including the POP tend to mask the menopause, it is not always necessary to know the precise time of final ovarian failure. Moreover, FSH levels are unreliable for diagnosis of complete loss of ovarian function. So one of the options in the box should be followed.

Plan A Contraception may cease: after waiting for the 'officially approved' 1yr of amenorrhoea above age 50, having stopped all hormones

This is the obvious plan for:
- copper IUDs.
- condoms.
- sponge or spermicides (which unlike in younger women appear to be adequate in the presence of such drastically reduced if not absent fertility).

But what to do if the woman is using one of the other hormonal methods or HRT, which mask the menopause?
- If on DMPA or COC (or Evra® patch): age 50 is the time to stop these (and maybe switch to a POP). They are needlessly strong, contraceptively, and the known risks increase with age.
- The POP, or an implant, or the LNG-IUS, or a sponge/spermicide with ongoing HRT: as contraceptives these add negligible medical risks that increase with age.

Therefore, one of these (usually the POP) may be continued until the latest age of potential fertility has been reached: then the woman just stops the contraception. When is that?
- A good estimate is age 55. The Faculty of FP in their guidance[1] quote Treloar's evidence that 95.9% have ceased menstruation for ever by then (and such bleeds as may happen later, in the other 4.1%, would be extremely unlikely to occur in cycles that were fertile).

Plan B Contraception may cease: at age 55 after having switched to, or having continued till then using a progestogen-only method—most commonly a POP (old type)
- There is also the option, especially if regular cycles return after stopping the POP even at age 55, simply to use a sponge or spermicide until final amenorrhoea is established.

Plan C Contraception may cease: above age 50 if three other criteria apply

Older users of hormonal contraception may cease using any method **IF**:
1. They have passed their 50th birthday, **AND**, after a trial of 2 months' discontinuation using barriers or spermicides, they have:
2. Vasomotor symptoms
3. Two separate high FSH levels (>30U/L) one month apart when off all treatment, and
4. Continuing amenorrhoea thereafter beyond this trial period.

With due warnings of lack of certainty, these women may cease all contraception earlier than the approved one year post-50. Or, as before, just use a sponge or spermicide until one year of time amenorrhoea is finally established.

1 FFPRHC Guidance (January 2005). Contraception for women aged over 40 years. *J Fam Plann Reprod Health Care* 1995; **31**: 51–63.

Appendix

☀ Use of licensed products in an unlicensed way

Often licensing procedures have not yet caught up with what is widely considered the best evidence-based practice. Such off-licence use is legitimate and may indeed be necessary for optimal contraceptive care, provided certain criteria are observed. These are well established.

The prescribing physician must

- Be adopting an evidence-based practice endorsed by a responsible body of professional opinion.
- **Assess the individual's priorities and preferences**, giving a clear account of known and possible risks and the benefits.
- **Explain to her that it is an unlicensed prescription**.
- **Obtain informed (verbal) consent and record this**.
- Ensure good practice, including follow-up, to comply fully with professional indemnity requirements: along with meticulous record-keeping.
- **NB: this will often mean the doctor providing dedicated written materials**, because the manufacturer's PIL insert may not apply in one or more respects.

This protocol is generally termed 'named-patient' prescribing.

Note that:
- Attention to detail is important, as in the (unlikely) event of a claim, the manufacturer can be excused from any liability.
- Independent nurse prescribers cannot *prescribe* medicines outside the terms of the licence, but they may supply and administer them as above within fully agreed and authorized Patient Group Directions or, as Supplementary Nurse Prescribers, prescribe within a Clinical Management Plan.

Some common examples of named-patient prescribing

- Advising more than the usual dosage, e.g. when EIDs are being used with:
  - the COC or POP or
  - hormonal emergency contraception.
- Sustained use of COC over many cycles:
  - long-term tricycling or, as now also proposed:
  - 365/365 use
- Use of banded copper IUDs for longer than licensed:
  - under the age of 40 (eg T-Safe™ Cu 380A for >10yrs, Nova T™ 380 for >5yrs) and
  - continuing use to postmenopause of *any* copper device that was fitted after age 40.
- Continuing use of the same LNG-IUS for contraception:
  - in an older woman (e.g. where fitted above 35) for up to 7yrs rather than the licensed 4, at a patient's fully informed request; and
  - indefinitely if fitted above 45 and she is amenorrhoeic (advice of NICE).
- Use of hormonal EC:

- beyond 72h after the earliest exposure, or
- more than once in a cycle.
- *Use of 'Quick Start'* This means, with appropriate safeguards (including applying the criteria on 📖 p. 430–31 to reduce conception risk), commencement of pills or other medical methods of contraception:
  - late in the menstrual cycle or
  - immediately after hormonal EC.

There are other examples you may identify elsewhere in this book.

Essential websites in reproductive health

www.ippf.org.uk
Online version of the *Directory of Hormonal Contraception*, with names of (equivalent) pill brands used throughout the world.

www.who.int/reproductive-health
WHO Medical Eligibility Criteria (WHOMEC) and new Practice Recommendations (WHOSPR).

www.ffprhc.org.uk
Includes UK-adapted Medical Eligibility Criteria (UKMEC), detailed Faculty of FP guidance on numerous contraceptive topics and also access to the invaluable *Journal of the Faculty of Family Planning and Reproductive Health Care*.

www.rcog.org.uk
Evidence-based Royal College Guidelines on male and female sterilization, infertility and menorrhagia.

www.nice.org.uk/guidance/CG30
Specific URL for valuable guidance from NICE on long-acting reversible contraceptives, 2005.

www.fertilityuk.org
The fertility awareness and NFP service, including teachers available.
Locally—a brilliant website, factual and non-sectarian.

www.bashh.org
National guidelines for the management of all STIs and contact details for GUM clinics throughout the UK.

www.fpa.org.uk
Patient information plus those essential leaflets! There is also an invaluable Helpline: 0845 310 1334.

www.brook.org.uk
Similar to the fpa website but for under 25s; plus a really secure online enquiry service. Helpline: 0800 0185023.

www.likeitis.org.uk
Reproductive health for lay persons by Marie Stopes. Brilliantly teenage friendly and matter-of-factual.

www.the-bms.org
Research-based advice about the menopause and HRT.

www.ipm.org.uk
Website of the Institute of Psychosexual Medicine.

www.basrt.org.uk
Website of the British Association for Sexual and Relationship Therapy; provides a list of therapists.

www.relate.org.uk
Enter postcode to get nearest Relate centre for relationship counselling and psychosexual therapy. Many publications are also available.
(Above three websites all give useful insights through their slightly differing approaches to psychosexual problems).

www.ecotimecapsule.com
John Guillebaud's website regarding population and the environment, plus 'Apology to the Future' project—and related sites:
www.optimumpopulation.org
www.populationandsustainability.org
www.popconnect.org – source of the dramatic DVD 'Population Dots'.
www.ruthinking.co.uk
Sex—are you thinking about it enough? Factual website that fully informs plus helps teens to access services in own local area. Supported by the Teenage Pregnancy Unit. Also Sexwise Helpline: 0800 282930

Further reading and references

Guillebaud J. Contraception—Your Questions Answered. Edinburgh: Churchill-Livingstone, 2004.

Guillebaud J. Contraception. In: McPherson A, Waller D, eds. Women's Health, 5th edn. Oxford: Oxford University Press, 2003 (formerly Women's Problems in General Practice).

National Institute for Health and Clinical Excellence. The effective and appropriate use of long-acting reversible contraception. London: RCOG, October 2005.
www.nice.org.uk/pdf/CG030fullguideline.pdf

WHO. Medical Eligibility Criteria for Contraceptive Use (WHOMEC). Geneva: WHO, 2004.

WHO. Selected Practice Recommendations for Contraceptive Use (WHOSPR). Geneva: WHO, 2005.

See www.who.int/reproductive-health for both of these.

More useful than WHOMEC in the UK is the UK adaptation known as UKMEC—see www.ffprhc.org.uk

Index